MRCS Revision Guide: Trunk and Thorax

D1330545

MRCS Revision Guide: Trunk and Thorax

Mazyar Kanani, MBBS, BSc, PhD, FRCS
Fellow in Congenital Cardiac Surgery, Children's Hospital, Pittsburgh, Pennsylvania, USA

Leanne Harling, MBBS, BSc, MRCS
Clinical Research Fellow, Department of Surgery and Cancer, Imperial College London, UK

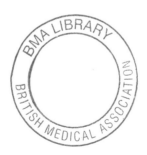

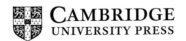

CAMBRIDGE UNIVERSITY PRESS
Cambridge, New York, Melbourne, Madrid, Cape Town,
Singapore, São Paulo, Delhi, Tokyo, Mexico City

Cambridge University Press
The Edinburgh Building, Cambridge CB2 8RU, UK

Published in the United States of America by
Cambridge University Press, New York

www.cambridge.org
Information on this title: www.cambridge.org/9780521145510

First published 2012

Printed in the United Kingdom at the University Press, Cambridge

A catalogue record for this publication is available from the British Library

Library of Congress Cataloguing-in-Publication Data

Kanani, Mazyar.
    MRCS revision guide: trunk and thorax / Mazyar Kanani, Leanne Harling.
        p. ; cm.
    Includes bibliographical references and index.
    ISBN 978-0-521-14551-0 (Paperback)
    I. Harling, Leanne.   II. Title.
    [DNLM: 1. Surgical Procedures, Operative–Examination Questions.   2. Surgical
Procedures, Operative–Outlines.   3. Thoracic Surgical Procedures–Examination
Questions.   4. Thoracic Surgical Procedures–Outlines.   WO 18.2]
    LC classification not assigned
    617′.9076–dc23   2011030676

ISBN 978-0-521-14551-0 Paperback

For my sister, Laura

For Robyn Eloise Caoimhe Kanani

Contents

Preface

In the face of the changing style of the intercollegiate MRCS examination, 'older' revision texts are no longer up to date with the novel exam format. In writing this book we aim to preserve the 'Socratic' method of question-and-answer that has previously been so well received amongst candidates. At the same time, we draw on our own personal experiences, of those students we have taught, and of those that have taught us, providing a novel text based on what you really need to know.

By combining a systems-based approach with the related anatomy and physiology, we hope that this book will not only act as a quick reference guide during a night on call, but also improve your overall understanding of each topic, providing that background information that we so greatly crave but often have insufficient time to search for.

We wish you the best of luck, not only in your exams, but also in the many years of surgical training that lie ahead.

Leanne Harling, Mazyar Kanani, 2011

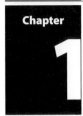

Chapter

Clinical surgery in general

Suture materials

What different types of suture do you know of?

Suture materials may be categorized as (1) natural, synthetic and metallic, (2) absorbable or non-absorbable, or (3) monofilament or multifilament.

Give examples of natural, synthetic and metallic sutures and their uses

Natural sutures

Catgut	Not used as has been banned in Europe and Japan, owing to concerns about transmission of prion disease.
Silk	General soft tissue closure and ligation. Avoid in vascular anastamoses and skin closure, owing to formation of stitch sinuses and abscesses.

Synthetic sutures

Vicryl/Vicryl Rapide (polyglactin)	Bowel anastamoses.
PDS (polydioxanone)	Mass closure of midline laparotomy incision.
Proline (polypropylene)	Closure of facial wounds and vascular anastamoses.
Ethilon (nylon, polyamide)	In ligation or general soft tissue approximation.

Metallic sutures

Steel	Closure of the sternum after median sternotomy.

How would you classify sutures according to absorbability?

Absorbable	Vicryl/Vicryl Rapide, PDS, catgut.
Non-absorbable	Prolene, nylon, silk, steel.

Over what period do the absorbable sutures degenerate?

Vicryl –– Complete absorption at 56–70 days. Retains 40% of its tensile strength at 4 weeks.

Vicryl Rapide –– Complete absorption at 42 days. Retains 0% of its tensile strength at 10–14 days.

PDS –– Completely hydrolyzed at 182–238 days. Retains 35–60% of its tensile strength at 6 weeks (depending on size of suture).

Chromic catgut –– Full tensile strength remains for 7–10 days and is fully hydrolyzed at 90 days. Pure catgut is absorbed more quickly and causes an intense tissue reaction.

Give examples of monofilament and multifilament sutures

Monofilament –– PDS, prolene, nylon.

Multifilament –– Vicryl or Vicryl Rapide, silk, catgut.

What are the advantages and disadvantages of monofilament sutures?

Advantages –– Less tissue reaction; glides easily; infection is less likely to settle in between the filaments, as may occur with braided sutures; less platelet activation (ideal for vascular anastamoses).

Disadvantages –– Monofilament sutures often have memory and can be difficult to handle and tie; requiring more throws to form a secure knot.

Summarize the sizing of suture materials

Suture sizes are defined by the United States Pharmacopeia (USP) scale. This scale uses zero as the baseline. As the suture diameter decreases below the baseline, zeros are added (e.g., 0000 or 4-0). As the suture diameter increases above the baseline, a number is given to denote the size (e.g., number 4). The smallest available suture is 11-0 (0.01 mm diameter) and is used in microsurgery and ophthalmology. The largest is a braided number 5 suture (0.7 mm diameter), which is often used in orthopaedics.

What types of needle are available? Give examples

Needles may be straight, curved or J-shaped. These may then be further categorized according to the body and the point of the needle. The body may be cutting, reverse-cutting or round-bodied. The point may be cutting, blunt or tapered. A forward-cutting needle has the sharp edge on the inside of the curve and a reverse-cutting needle has the cutting edge on the outside (preventing inside cut-out). Round-bodied, blunt needles are used in tissues that may be easily penetrated and damaged (e.g., in mass closure of abdominal midline laparotomy incisions, to prevent damage to the underlying bowel).

Diathermy

What different types of diathermy are available?

Monopolar (cutting, coagulation and blend) and bipolar (coagulation only). Both use alternating current (ac).

Give examples of uses of each

Monopolar diathermy is used in most general surgical procedures. Cutting diathermy may be used on dissection though soft tissues, whereas coagulation is often used on small vessels. Bipolar diathermy is used in extremity surgery to prevent high current densities over a small area of tissue (e.g., fingers). It is also used in neurosurgical and plastic surgical procedures, where finer precision is required.

What is the difference between monopolar and bipolar diathermy?

Monopolar -- A high current density is produced at the tip of the diathermy probe, which then disseminates throughout the body as it is conducted to the diathermy plate (or indifferent electrode). To reduce the current density at the diathermy plate and prevent a heating effect, the diathermy plate must have a minimum surface area of 70 cm^2. Incorrect placement of the plate or contact with other conducting materials may result in burns. Power used is up to 400 W.

Bipolar -- The diathermy instrument consists of two electrodes (commonly combined as forceps) and current is conducted between the two electrodes; it only passes through the tissue that is being treated. It uses significantly lower power than monopolar diathermy and there is no need for a diathermy plate. Cutting is not possible with bipolar diathermy. Power used is up to 50 W.

Why does surgical diathermy not produce muscle stimulation?

The high frequency of current in the diathermy circuit prevents muscle stimulation unless applied directly to striated muscle. The frequency of current used by diathermy units is 400 kHz to 10 MHz (mains frequency is 50 kHz). Muscle stimulation is produced at frequencies of <50 kHz and at this frequency even small currents (5–10 mA) may cause muscle stimulation. The use of higher frequencies therefore also allows much higher currents to be safely conducted through tissues.

What is the difference between the cutting and coagulation settings?
What other settings may be used?

Cutting -- A continuous current output allows arcing of the current between the tip of the electrode and the tissue. This creates a temperature of approximately 1000 °C in the local tissue, resulting in vaporization of cell water and tissue disruption. There is little coagulation when this setting is used.

Coagulation –– A pulsed current output is generated, resulting in local heat production with tissue desiccation and sealing of blood vessels. There is minimal tissue disruption.

Other available settings include fulguration (spray coagulation) and blend. Fulguration uses a high voltage to coagulate over a wider area. Blend produces a continuous output with pulses that allows simultaneous coagulation and cutting.

What are the risks associated with diathermy?

1. Incorrect plate position may result in burns, owing to poor heat dissipation. The plate must be positioned over areas with good blood supply and away from bony prominences, scar tissue and metal implants.

2. Bowel gas and alcoholic skin preparations that are not sufficiently allowed to dry may result in explosion.

3. There is potential for diathermy smoke to contain carcinogens. Direct inhalation should be avoided.

4. Use of monopolar diathermy on appendages may result in setting up high current density locally (without the ability to dissipate current), causing tissue damage distant from the site of the electrode.

5. The use of diathermy adjacent to metal implants or other metal objects may allow current to be induced in a metal object without direct contact between it and the diathermy electrode. This could result in heating around the metal object and tissue damage.

6. Capacitance coupling: the diathermy electrode comprises a metal active wire surrounded by an insulating layer. In laparoscopic surgery, this is then contained within a metal cannula, which passes through a port (either metal or plastic) into the abdominal cavity. In this set-up, ac current may be conducted from the active wire to the surrounding metal cannula without direct contact, as the insulating layer acts as the capacitor. The stray current is then dissipated through the patient's body to the diathermy plate, provided that the cannula is housed within a metal port. The current density is usually low and little or no heating effect occurs around the port site. If however, a metal cannula is used with a non-conducting port there will be no discharge current from the cannula before its entry into the abdominal cavity. This may result in damage to structures (e.g., the bowel) that are in contact with the cannula but out of view.

7. Direct coupling: if the electrode is in contact with another metal object, this will result in conduction of current through this object and may cause heating and damage to adjacent tissues.

What are the relative contraindications to the use of diathermy?

Pacemakers or implantable cardiac defibrillators (ICDs). Monopolar diathermy should be avoided where possible, as it may cause:

1. Induced current down the pacemaker wires, resulting in myocardial burns.
2. Induced currents in the pacemaker unit resulting in potential change to pacing rate or inhibition of output. An ICD may be inappropriately stimulated, owing to misinterpretation of an interference signal as myocardial activity. Both these instances may result in fatal arrhythmias.

Which measures may be taken to reduce the risks when using diathermy in patients with pacemakers or ICDs?

1. Avoid monopolar diathermy: use only bipolar diathermy devices.
2. Avoid the use of cutting diathermy.
3. Where coagulation diathermy is used, this should only be in short bursts.
4. The active electrode and diathermy plate should be positioned as far as possible from the thorax.
5. The thorax should not form part of the current path.
6. External pacing should be available for emergency use in the case of pacemaker malfunction.

Skin preparation and asepsis

What different types of skin preparation solutions are you aware of?

The solutions most commonly used are:

10% Povidone-iodine –– Bactericidal as well as bacteriostatic, with little irritation to skin or mucosa. It can be used as a skin preparation solution and in areas where the skin is breached.

Chlorhexidine 0.5% in 70% alcohol –– Bactericidal and bacteriostatic, although reduced bactericidal effect with some gram-negative bacteria. Care should be taken to allow alcohol preparation solutions to dry before the use of electrocautery, as there is a risk that vapour may ignite.

What are the most commonly used surgical scrub solutions?

Povidone-iodine 7.5% (Betadine) and Chlorhexidine gluconate 4%.

What is the difference between sterilization and disinfection?

Sterilization is defined as a process by which all microorganisms (bacteria, fungi and viruses) are destroyed. Disinfection is a process in which infective microorganisms are removed (bacteria, fungi and viruses).

What are the different methods of sterilization?

Steam (via autoclave) –– Autoclaves produce moist heat, combining temperature and pressure. Requirements to achieve sterilization are 134 °C for 3 min at 2 kPa or 121 °C for 15 min at 1 kPa. Autoclaving does not necessarily eliminate prions (usually treated with sodium hydroxide for 2 hours plus autoclaving for 1 hour at 160 °C).

Dry heat –– Requires much longer duration than moist heat, used for moisture-sensitive objects. Requirements for sterilization are at least 2 hours at 160 °C or 6–12 minutes at 190 °C.

Ethylene oxide –– Used in heat-sensitive objects: it kills all known bacteria, spores, fungi and viruses. The disadvantages are that it requires a longer period of sterilization, requires poststerilization aeration to remove toxic residues and is highly flammable.

Peracetic acid (0.2%) –– Used in sterilization of endoscopes.

Radiation –– Gamma radiation is used for industrial sterilization of instruments and other equipment (cannulae, syringes, giving sets, etc.). Not used on a small scale, owing to the requirements for housing and safe use of gamma radioisotopes.

What systems are in place in the operating theatre to reduce the risk of infection?

Laminar flow operating rooms –– Air cycles with a minimum of 300 changes per hour. Used in orthopaedic theatres to reduce the risk of implant infection (a fourfold reduction has been shown in studies).

Positive pressure ventilation –– Approximately 20 changes per hour. Higher pressure in the clean areas and lower pressure in the dirty areas results in flow of air from clean to dirty areas. This reduces the bacterial count in clean areas.

Laparoscopy: the basics

What techniques do you know to achieve pneumoperitoneum?

Hasson technique (open) –– Recommended by the Royal College of Surgeons. Make an infraumbilical incision of approximately 1–2 cm. Dissect through subcutaneous tissues until reaching the linea alba. Make an incision in the linea alba and place either a purse string or stay sutures around the incision. Continue to dissect through the extraperitoneal fat until the peritoneum is visualized. Make a 1–2 cm incision in the peritoneum and under direct vision introduce a 10 mm camera port with the sharp trocar removed (or use a blunt-tipped trocar). Insufflate the peritoneum with carbon dioxide. A low pressure with high flow indicates correct positioning of the port within the peritoneal cavity. Aim for a pressure of 12–14 mmHg (can preset).

Veress needle (blind) –– A small infraumbilical incision should be made and the Veress needle carefully inserted through the deeper structures, directed towards the coccyx. A 'pop' is usually felt as the needle passes through the linea alba and peritoneum. Various methods are used to confirm pneumoperitoneum; the commonest is the 'saline drop test'. A drop of saline placed at the Veress needle bulb is immediately sucked into the needle as it is inserted through the peritoneum, owing to the negative intra-abdominal pressure.

OptiView ports –– These are an alternative method of obtaining a 'closed' pneumoperitoneum. The laparoscope is inserted into the 12 mm trocar as it is advanced into the peritoneal cavity. The tip of the trocar is transparent, allowing direct visualization of each tissue layer as it is traversed. The peritoneal cavity is therefore entered under direct vision and the length of the incision made is minimized.

What are the complications associated with pneumoperitoneum?

Respiratory –– High intra-abdominal pressure may result in diaphragmatic splinting and hence reduce pulmonary compliance, leading to ventilation–perfusion mismatch, reducing gaseous exchange. Carbon dioxide insufflation can lead to hypercapnia and respiratory acidosis. High ventilation pressures used to compensate for high insufflation pressures may lead to barotrauma and pneumothorax.

Cardiovascular –– Raised intra-abdominal pressure reduces venous return (worsened by head-up positioning) resulting in a reduction in cardiac output. The subsequent venous stasis as a result of a reduction in venous return may increase the incidence of thromboembolism.

General
1. Gas embolism, either due to inadvertent venepuncture with Veress needle or, infrequently, as a direct result of intraperitoneal gas pressure,
2. Visceral puncture.
3. Insufflation of the omentum.

What are the advantages and disadvantages of laparoscopic surgery over open surgery?

Advantages –– Smaller incisions; less postoperative pain; decreased incidence of wound complications; shorter hospital stay; earlier return to work; improved cosmesis; reduced adhesion formation (although similar rates of adhesion-related complications have been seen with laparoscopic gynaecological surgery).[1]

Disadvantages –– Inadvertent damage to surrounding structures due to limited view of operating field; reduced tactile feedback; not suitable for all patients; steep learning curve.

What are the contraindications to laparoscopic surgery?

Relative –– Clotting abnormalities; deranged liver function; cardiac failure; raised intracranial pressure; respiratory dysfunction; generalized peritonitis; obliteration of the intraperitoneal space (e.g., due to adhesions, organomegaly, reoperation and pregnancy).

Absolute –– Uncontrolled shock; intestinal obstruction.

[1] A. M. Lower, R. J. S. Hawthorn, H. Ellis *et al.* (2000). The impact of adhesions on hospital readmissions over ten years after 8849 open gynaecological operations: an assessment from the Surgical and Clinical Adhesions Research Study. *Br. J. Obstet. Gynaecol.* **107**:855–862.

Applied surgical anatomy

2

What is the anatomical position of the heart within the chest?

The heart is located in the middle mediastinum and is covered anteriorly by the costal cartilages of the third, fourth and fifth ribs.

Describe the reflections of the pericardium and describe the location of the transverse and oblique sinuses

The pericardium is made up of a visceral layer, which is adherent to the heart, and a parietal layer, which forms the inner surface of the pericardial sac. There is a small amount of serous pericardial fluid between the two layers. There are two recesses within the pericardium: the transverse sinus and the oblique sinus. The transverse sinus is bounded anteriorly by the posterior surface of the aorta and the pulmonary trunk and posteriorly by the anterior surface of the interatrial groove. The oblique sinus is the space behind the left atrium and is bounded by the pericardial reflections of the inferior vena cava and the pulmonary veins.

What is meant by coronary artery dominance?

Dominance is determined by the artery supplying the posterior descending artery (PDA). Approximately 85% of the population are right coronary dominant (PDA supplied by the right coronary artery), and 10% are left dominant (PDA supplied by the circumflex artery). Co-dominance is seen in the remaining 5%.

Briefly describe the course of the right coronary artery

The right coronary artery arises from the anterior aortic sinus between the right atrium and the pulmonary trunk. It descends in the right atrioventricular groove supplying the right atrium and ventricle before reaching the inferior border of the heart where it gives off an acute marginal branch and, in 85% of the population, the posterior descending artery (PDA). The PDA continues to the apex, where it anastamoses with the corresponding branch of the left coronary artery.

What are the key branches of the right coronary artery?

The (sino-atrial) nodal artery –– The blood supply to the sino-atrial node is from the RCA in approximately 60% of individuals.

The atrioventricular nodal artery –– This arises from the RCA in approximately 85% of the population. The RCA then gives rise to a marginal artery and the posterior descending artery (posterior intraventricular artery) in approximately 85% (see note on dominance) of the population.

Briefly describe the course of the left coronary artery and its branches

The left coronary artery arises as the left mainstem from the posterior (left) aortic sinus and passes posterior and to the left of the pulmonary trunk. It then bifurcates to form the circumflex and left anterior descending arteries.

Briefly describe the structure and position of the aortic valve

The surface marking of the aortic valve is the left sternal edge in the third intercostal space (ICS). The normal aortic valve has three cup-shaped cusps and lies within the bulge of the proximal aorta. The aortic sinuses prevent the cusps being flattened against the wall of the aorta during ventricular systole and allow blood flow into the sinuses during diastole. This in turn distends the cusps, forcing them together and closing the valve.

Briefly describe the structure and position of the mitral valve

The surface marking of the mitral valve is the fourth costal cartilage at the left sternal edge. The mitral valve is a bicuspid valve, made up of a fibrous annulus, the anterior and posterior leaflets, the chordae tendinae and the papillary muscles.

What is the anatomical position of the sino-atrial node (SAN)?

The SAN lies at the junction between the right atrium and the superior vena cava at the anterior and superior extent of the terminal groove. It is usually to the right or lateral of the superior cavo-atrial junction.

What is the blood supply to the SAN?

In approximately 60% of people, the SAN is supplied by the nodal artery, which is a branch of the right coronary artery. In the remaining 40%, it arises from a branch of the circumflex artery. From its origin, it usually runs along the anterior interatrial groove to the position of the SAN at the superior cavo-atrial junction.

What is the anatomical position of the atrioventricular node (AVN)?

It occupies the upper part of Koch's triangle. Koch's triangle is bounded by the septal leaflet of the tricuspid valve, the ostium of the coronary sinus and the tendon of Todaro. The tendon of Todaro is a fibrous structure formed by the junction of the eustachian valve (within the inferior vena cava) and the thebesian valve (within the coronary sinus).

What is the anatomical position of the bundle of His?

The bundle of His is located at the apex of Koch's triangle. It travels from the apex of Koch's triangle along the intraventricular septum, where it then branches.

Describe the course of the phrenic nerve as it runs through the thoracic cavity

The phrenic nerve originates from the C3, C4 and C5 nerve roots and runs in the neck to enter the thoracic cavity via the thoracic inlet. Here it lies on the surface of the scalenus anterior along with the internal mammary artery. After entry into the thoracic cavity, the course of the nerve is different on either side. On the right, it runs anterior to the brachiocephalic artery and posterior to the subclavian vein. It then courses along with the lateral edge of the superior vena cava and runs anterior to the hilum of the lung. It finally passes through the vena caval hiatus of the diaphragm (T8), where it then branches onto and supplies the right hemidiaphragm. On the left, it descends anterior to the subclavian artery and aortic arch. It then runs on the anterior surface of the pericardial sac along the obtuse margin of the heart to pierce the diaphragm independently. It does not pass through any of the diaphragmatic openings. It eventually branches onto (and supplies) the left hemidiaphragm.

Describe the course of the vagus nerve as it runs through the thoracic cavity

The vagus nerve arises from the medulla oblongata and exits the skull base through the jugular foramen. It then passes in the carotid sheath in the neck between the carotid artery and the internal jugular vein. After entering the thoracic cavity, its course varies on either side. The right vagus lies in direct contact with the trachea. It passes anterior to the subclavian artery and gives off the recurrent laryngeal nerve before descending posterior to the SVC. It then passes posterior to the hilum of the lung, giving off the branches of the pulmonary plexus. From here, it follows the oesophagus through the oesophageal opening of the diaphragm at the level of T10, where its terminal branches form the posterior oesophageal plexus. The left vagus passes between the subclavian artery and the innominate vein before giving off the left recurrent laryngeal nerve. It then runs posterior to the hilum of the lung giving off branches to the pulmonary plexus and travels anteriorly on the oesophagus, through the oesophageal hiatus of the diaphragm, to form the anterior oesophageal plexus.

Explain the differing course of the recurrent laryngeal nerve on each side, and its embryological significance

The right recurrent laryngeal nerve is given off at the thoracic inlet and loops around the right subclavian artery before ascending into the neck. The left recurrent laryngeal nerve loops posteriorly around the ligamentum arteriosum (aortic arch) before ascending into the neck in the tracheo-oesophageal groove. This difference is a result of the embryological development of the aortic arches. In the embryo, the truncus arteriosus arises from the bulbus cordis to give rise to six pairs of aortic arches. During development, the first and second arches disappear and the third becomes the carotids. The fourth becomes the brachiocephalic and subclavian artery on the right, but on the left, it becomes the aortic arch and gives off the subclavian. The fifth disappears and the sixth forms the pulmonary arteries. On the left, the sixth arch remains in connection with the dorsal aorta by means of the ductus arteriosus. On the right side, as the fifth and distal sixth arches disappear, the recurrent laryngeal nerve hooks around fourth arch – the subclavian artery. On the left, the nerve remains hooked around the ligamentum arteriosum – the remaining distal part of the sixth arch.

Describe the surface markings of the lungs and pleura

Pleurae –– Both pleurae extend approximately 2.5 cm above the clavicle. They then pass behind the level of the sternoclavicular joint to meet medially at the level of the angle of Louis (second costal cartilage). From here, the left pleura reflects around the heart and the right descends vertically to the sixth costal cartilage. Both pleurae then cross the eighth rib at the midclavicular line, the tenth rib at the midaxillary line and the twelfth rib posteriorly at the lateral border of the erector spinae.

Lungs –– The exact extent of the lungs varies during the respiratory cycle. Their position is approximately two rib spaces different from that of the pleura. Each lung crosses the sixth rib at the midclavicular line, the eighth rib at the midaxillary line and the tenth rib posteriorly at the lateral border of the erector spinae.

At which sites are the pleurae at risk surgically?

Above the clavicle –– The pleurae extend 2.5 cm above the clavicle and may be injured during central venous line insertion.

At the level of the twelfth rib –– The pleurae may be injured during nephrectomy as they descend just below the twelfth rib posteromedially.

What are the surface markings of the lung fissures?

The oblique fissure –– This divides the lung into the upper and lower lobes. Its position can be drawn along the medial border of the scapula with the shoulder fully abducted. Alternatively, in the anatomical position it corresponds to a line extending from a point 2.5 cm lateral to the spine of the fifth thoracic vertebra obliquely downwards to the sixth costal cartilage, 4 cm from the midline.

The horizontal fissure –– This separates the middle and upper lobes of the right lung. It corresponds to a horizontal line along the fourth costal cartilage, where it meets the line of the oblique fissure at the level of the fifth rib.

Briefly describe the segmentation of bronchi

The right main bronchus –– This further divides into the upper, middle and lower lobe bronchi. The upper lobe bronchus has three further subdivisions (apical, posterior and anterior), the middle has two (lateral and medial) and the lower has two (apical and basal).

The left main bronchus –– This further divides into the upper, lingular and lower lobe bronchi. The upper lobe bronchus has two subdivisions (apicoposterior and anterior), the lingular has two (superior and inferior), and the lower has two (apical and basal).

Briefly describe the blood supply to the lung and bronchi

The pulmonary arteries return mixed venous blood to the lungs, where it is oxygenated. The arterial supply to the bronchi is via the bronchial arteries. The pulmonary veins (superior and inferior) return oxygenated blood to the left atrium. The venous drainage of the bronchi is via the bronchial veins, which drain into the azygous vein, which in turn drains into the SVC.

Which key structures can be identified in a plane at the angle of Louis? To what vertebral level does this correspond?

The angle of Louis (sterno-manubrial junction) is at the level of the second rib anteriorly. This corresponds to the level of the T4/T5 intervertebral disc posteriorly. The structures identified at this level are:

1. The carina (bifurcation of the trachea),
2. The beginning and end of the aortic arch,
3. The azygous vein joins the SVC,
4. The division of the pulmonary trunk,
5. The ligamentum arteriosum,
6. The cardiac plexuses,
7. The thoracic duct crosses from right to left (it then ascends into the neck to enter the venous system at the junction of the left internal jugular and left subclavian veins).

Applied surgical physiology: cardiovascular

Important equations in cardiac physiology

What is the definition of cardiac output?

Cardiac output (CO) is the amount of blood ejected by the heart in one minute. It is equal to the product of the heart rate (HR) and the stroke volume (SV):

$$CO = HR \times SV$$

What is the definition of stroke volume?

This is the volume of blood ejected by the heart in one cardiac cycle.

What is the normal resting value for cardiac output?

$$5 - 6 \ l/min$$

What is the relationship between CO, systemic vascular resistance (SVR) and blood pressure (BP)?

$$BP = CO \times SVR$$

What factors influence stroke volume?

Preload, afterload, heart rate and myocardial contractility.

Define preload

This is the volume of blood returning to the heart, i.e., it is the venous return. The volume of venous return is the difference between the systemic filling pressure and the central venous pressure.

Define afterload

Afterload is the ventricular wall tension that has to be generated in order to eject blood out of the ventricle. It is analogous to the arterial pressure. It is equal to the product of the cardiac output and the systemic vascular resistance (SVR):

$$Afterload = CO \times SVR$$

Increasing cardiac output increases arterial pressure, and so has a negative feedback effect on cardiac output due to the increased afterload. More energy is consumed generating enough pressure to overcome the arterial pressure, therefore there is a reduction in the stroke volume and a resultant reduction in cardiac output.

Starling's law of the heart

What is the Frank–Starling relationship? Can you draw a curve to represent this?

Frank–Starling's law states that the greater the end diastolic volume (volume of blood entering the heart during diastole), the greater the stroke volume (volume of blood ejected during systole) and vice versa. Figure 3.1 demonstrates this.

What is meant by excitation–contraction coupling?

This is the process by which the arrival of an action potential (AP) causes a myocyte to contract. The arrival of the AP causes an influx of calcium ions through L-type calcium channels in the sarcolemma. Further calcium release is then triggered from the sarcoplasmic reticulum. This free calcium activates troponin C, which induces a conformational change in troponin I, such that a site on the actin molecule is exposed allowing the myosin head to bind. The hydrolysis of ATP by the myosin head ATPase generates the energy for the 'ratcheting' of the myosin heads on the actin, shortening the sarcomere.

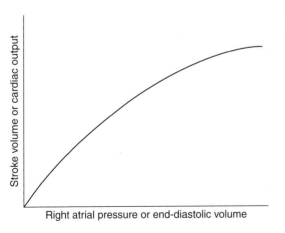

Figure 3.1 The Frank–Starling relationship.

Stroke volume or cardiac output

Right atrial pressure or end-diastolic volume

How does an increase in myocyte stretch generate an increase in cardiac output?

Myocyte stretch increases the sarcomere length, and this in turn increases troponin C calcium sensitivity. This increases the rate of cross bridge attachment and detachment and hence the tension developed by the muscle fibre.

Why does the cardiac output eventually fall at very high levels of stretch or of end diastolic volume?

The actin and myosin fibres no longer overlap, leading to loss of contraction.

What happens to the curve if the myocardial contractility is increased?

The curve shifts upwards. The stroke volume is higher for any given end diastolic volume.

What measures may be used to increase cardiac output?

| **Increasing contractility** | Inotropic agents – increase sympathetic stimulation. |
| **Decreasing afterload** | Vasodilators (e.g. GTN) – reduce systemic vascular resistance. |

Both of these will move the patient to a higher curve, i.e., there will be a higher stroke volume for any given myocardial stretch.

What is the physiological response to standing up?

Standing up leads to pooling of blood in the peripheries and hence decreases the venous return to the heart. By Starling's law, this results in a temporary reduction in cardiac output. As $BP = SVR \times CO$, this leads to a reduction in blood pressure. This fall in blood pressure is sensed by the baroreceptors in the aortic arch and carotid sinus, leading to a reflex constriction of the arterioles and capillaries. This increase in SVR results in a normalization of the blood pressure. Sympathetic stimulation caused by the fall in CO also results in a reflex tachycardia. In addition, the increase in sympathetic drive causes an increase in contractility.

How does this compare to the physiological response to the Valsalva manoeuvre?

The Valsalva manoeuvre is forced expiration against a closed glottis. This increases the intra-thoracic pressure and hence reduces venous return. This leads to the same cascade of physiological compensation as occurs when standing up. On releasing the manoeuvre, there is a recovery phase, leading to a rise in arterial pressure, which stimulates the baroreceptors and leads to a reflex bradycardia.

What is the practical use of testing the Valsalva manoeuvre?

It is used as a test for autonomic function. In patients with autonomic neuropathy, there is a sustained fall in arterial pressure throughout the manoeuvre. There is also no recovery phase.

The cardiac cycle and coronary circulation

Draw a diagram to represent the pressure changes in the left heart during the cardiac cycle. How does this relate to the ECG waveform?

See Figure 3.2.

What is meant by isovolumetric contraction?

This is the phase where the ventricle contracts without a change in volume. Both the aortic and mitral valves are closed, causing a sharp increase in the wall tension of the left ventricle but at constant volume. The rate of change in wall tension (dP/dt) can be used as a measure of myocardial contractility.

What is the significance of the dicrotic notch in the aortic pressure waveform?

This represents closure of the aortic valve. The momentum of blood flow across the aortic valve during ejection ensures continued flow into the aortic

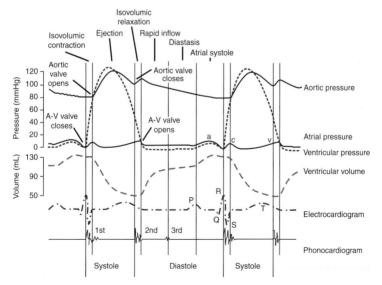

Figure 3.2 Pressure and volume changes in the left heart during the cardiac cycle, with ECG waveform.

root despite being against the pressure gradient. The eventual closure of the aortic valve is forceful and this leads to a brief rise in the pressure in the aortic root, producing the dicrotic notch.

What is meant by the 'atrial kick'? Which part of the graph represents this phenomenon?

Ventricular filling is predominantly a passive process, owing to the pressure difference between the atrium and ventricle on opening of the atrioventricular valve. At the end of this process, there is a final contraction of the atrium, known as the 'atrial kick'. This can be seen in Figure 3.2 as a brief rise in pressure in the atrium just prior to the onset of ventricular systole.

What is the mean arterial pressure (MAP)?

$$MAP = \text{Diastolic pressure} + \frac{1}{3}(\text{Systolic pressure} - \text{Diastolic pressure}).$$

MAP is not the mean of the systolic and diastolic pressures, as it is time weighted. For approximately two-thirds of the cardiac cycle, the pressure is closer to the diastolic pressure.

Draw a graph to represent the arterial pressure waveform

See Figure 3.3. The dicrotic notch represents closure of the aortic valve, as previously described.

How does the arterial pressure waveform vary throughout the arterial tree?

As blood travels away from the heart, the systolic pressure increases and the pulse pressure increases. The diastolic and mean arterial pressure decrease, but to a lesser extent. There is also a temporal delay in the systolic pressure

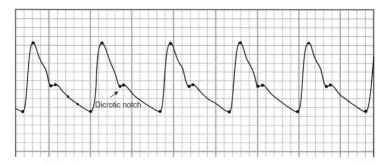

Figure 3.3 The arterial pressure waveform.

upstroke, reflecting the distance from the heart at which the pressure wave-form is measured (approximately 60 ms at the radial artery).

What is the reason for this variation?

1. The progressive increase in arterial wall stiffness, moving away from the heart (decreased compliance of the vessel wall).
2. The interaction between the transmitted and reflected waveforms, moving further away from the heart.

What are the homeostatic mechanisms that control blood pressure?

Blood pressure control may be divided into early (neural control), intermediate (renal control) and late (hormonal control) phases.

Baroreceptors –– These are found in the aortic arch and carotid sinus. They are pressure receptors from which sensory afferents are carried in the IX and X (glossopharyngeal and vagus) cranial nerves to the midbrain. From here, efferent sympathetic fibres lead to correction of the perceived change in blood pressure. This occurs via stimulation of the sympathetic nervous system and release of adrenaline and noradrenaline from the adrenal medulla, which acts directly on $\beta 1$ and $\beta 2$ receptors on the myocardium. This sympathetic stimulation also leads to peripheral vasoconstriction, an increase in SVR and an increase in blood pressure (BP = CO × SVR). The intermediate effect is a reduction in renal blood flow secondary to renal vasoconstriction and hence a reduction in GFR and a reduction in urine output. This consequentially leads to an increase in blood volume and hence an increase in blood pressure.

Renal and hormonal –– A fall in blood pressure is also sensed by the volume sensors in the right atrium (RA), leading to a reduction in atrial natriuretic peptide (ANP) production and hence a reduction of the secretion of ADH from the posterior lobe of the pituitary. This in turn increases the production of aquaporin 2 at the renal collecting duct and increases the reabsorption of water, increasing the blood volume and increasing the intravascular pressure. The reduction in renal arterial pressure (acutely below ~90 mmHg) stimulates the renin-angiotensin-aldosterone (R-A-A) system, which in turn leads to a cascade of effects to further increase in blood pressure.

Describe the cascade of effects involved in activation of the RAA system

A fall in blood pressure stimulates alpha-1 adrenoceptors, leading to an increase in renin production from the juxtaglomerular apparatus (JGA) of the kidney. This stimulates the conversion of angiotensinogen to angiotensin I, which is then converted to angiotensin II by angiotensin-converting

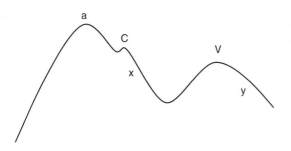

Figure 3.4 The central venous pressure waveform.

enzyme (ACE) produced by the lung. This process occurs approximately 30–60 minutes after the initial fall in BP. Angiotensin II stimulates aldosterone production from the adrenal cortex and the two hormones together act to cause vasoconstriction and a rise in BP. A secondary effect of angiotensin II is to stimulate the hypothalamus to further increase ADH production and stimulate thirst, so as to increase blood volume. Aldosterone also increases sodium reabsorption (and potassium secretion) in the renal tubules and hence water reabsorption.

Draw a diagram to represent the central venous pressure waveform

See Figure 3.4

What do the areas labelled in Figure 3.4 represent?

a Atrial contraction.

C Bulging of the tricuspid valve into the right atrium (RA) at the start of ventricular systole.

x The end of atrial systole.

V Progressive venous return into the RA, leading to a rise in the venous pressure. Its timing corresponds with ventricular systole.

y Opening of the tricuspid valve.

What is the normal range for central venous pressure (CVP)?

0 – 10 mmHg.

Note: It is the change in CVP that is important clinically and not just the absolute value. The CVP should be taken in the context of the overall status of the patient. For example, whilst small increases in CVP may result in a significant improvement in overall cardiac output when the patient is under-filled, if the plateau of cardiac function reserve is reached, further increases in CVP may lead to worsened haemodynamics.

What factors are important in determining CVP?

Blood volume –– Low circulating blood volume will lead to a low CVP.

Intra-thoracic pressure –– A more negative intra-thoracic pressure will lead to an increase in venous return to the heart (e.g., as occurs in inspiration) and hence CVP. The opposite occurs in expiration.

Skeletal muscle pump –– Mobilization leads to the contraction of the calf muscles and an increase in the venous return to the heart from the deep soleus plexus of veins.

Posture –– Elevation of the legs increases venous return and CVP.

Venous tone –– Venoconstriction via sympathetic stimulation leads to increased venous return and CVP.

The mechanics of breathing, ventilation and airway management

What are the indications for mechanical ventilation?

- Apnoea,
- Inadequate ventilation (tidal volume less than 5 ml/kg or vital capacity less than 10–15 ml/kg),
- Tachypnoea with imminent exhaustion (RR > 35),
- Decreased consciousness,
- Hypoxia refractory to oxygen therapy (P_aO_2 < 8 kPa with F_iO_2 > 0.6),
- Risk of obstruction or aspiration,
- Use in control of PCO_2 in head injury patients (keeping PCO_2 at 4.0–4.5 kPa reduces intracranial pressure by promoting cerebral vasoconstriction).

What is a definitive airway?

A tube present within the trachea (or bronchi if a double-lumen tube is used) with the cuff inflated, connected to oxygen-enriched assisted ventilation and secured in place.

Give examples of a definitive airway

- Endotracheal tube,
- Nasotracheal tube,
- Tracheostomy tube (cuff inflated, non-fenestrated).

In which situations should you consider placing a definitive airway?

Emergency
- Decreased consciousness,
- Any patient with an imminent risk of airway obstruction,

- Thermal injury (facial burns),
- Facial fractures,
- Direct airway injury,
- Stridor,
- Thoracic trauma, and
- Any emergency procedures where the patient is not adequately starved and there is a resulting high risk of aspiration.

Elective
- Complex or high-risk procedures where prolonged ventilation is likely to be required,
- Thoracic procedures where single lung ventilation may be necessary,
- Abdominal, facial and ENT surgery.

What are the basic modes of ventilation?

Pressure control –– The ventilator is set to produce a set pressure with each breath but, as a result, the generated tidal volume varies with lung compliance and resistance. Tidal and minute volume must be closely monitored.

Volume control –– A set tidal volume is delivered with each breath with constant inspiratory flow. This means that the airway pressure increases throughout inspiration, and tidal volume remains constant even with changes in lung compliance.

Controlled mandatory ventilation (CMV) –– The ventilator generates a set volume or pressure at a set rate. There is no allowance for spontaneous ventilation.

Synchronized intermittent mandatory ventilation (SIMV) –– Controlled breaths (either pressure or volume controlled) are generated at a preset respiratory rate, separately from any spontaneous breaths.

Pressure support ventilation (PSV) –– The patient breathes spontaneously and each breath stimulates the ventilator to generate a set amount of pressure, assisting each breath.

Which non-invasive methods of ventilation are available? Briefly describe the mechanisms by which they improve oxygenation

Continuous positive airways pressure (CPAP) –– This supplies a continuous positive pressure throughout the respiratory cycle and splints open alveoli. This improves recruitment and reduces the work of breathing, as it reduces the initial inspiratory effort needed to overcome the surface tension within the alveoli. It is especially useful in type 1 respiratory failure. However, the patient must be sufficiently conscious and compliant with the treatment.

Bi-level positive airways pressure (BIPAP) –– This provides two levels of positive pressure: inspiratory positive airways pressure (IPAP) and expiratory positive airways pressure (EPAP), and hence facilitates inspiration and expiration, decreasing the work of breathing. It is used in type 2 respiratory failure to improve hypoxia as well as to increase carbon dioxide removal.

Pressure support ventilation –– This monitors the patient's own ventilatory cycle and provides additional positive pressure when it senses inspiration.

What is PEEP?

Positive end expiratory pressure. Pressure delivered at the end of expiration splints open alveoli, improves compliance and recruitment and reduces the work of breathing. The pressure used is commonly 5–20 cmH$_2$O.

What are the complications of mechanical ventilation?

Respiratory –– Barotrauma: alveolar rupture as a result of high positive pressure may lead to spontaneous pneumothorax or pneumomediastinum.

Cardiovascular –– Venous return to the heart is augmented by negative pressure within the thoracic cavity. Positive pressure ventilation reduces this effect, hence reducing venous return to the heart and leading to an associated reduction in cardiac output and arterial pressure.

Renal –– A reduction in renal perfusion pressure may lead to a reduction in urine output.

Gastrointestinal –– An increased incidence of paralytic ileus has been associated with positive pressure ventilation.

Draw a basic spirometry trace and define the various parameters

See Figure 3.5.

Tidal volume (TV)	This is the volume of air displaced between normal inspiration and expiration when no forced effort is applied.
Functional residual capacity (FRC)	The volume of air present in the lungs at the end of passive expiration.
Total lung capacity	The volume of air contained within the lung at the end of maximal inspiration.
Residual volume (RV)	The volume of air left in the lungs at the end of maximal expiration.
Vital capacity (VC)	The volume between maximal inspiration and maximal expiration (this is the maximal volume that may be moved in and out of the lungs).

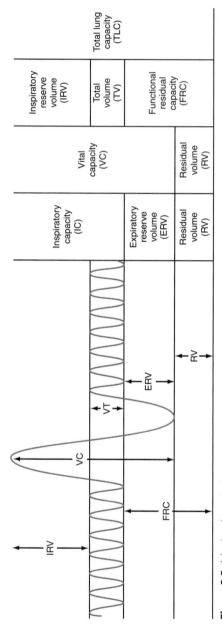

Figure 3.5 A basic spirometry trace.

| **Inspiratory reserve volume (IRV)** | The additional volume of air that may be inspired after normal inspiration. |
| **Expiratory reserve volume (ERV)** | The additional volume of air that may be expired after normal expiration. |

What is 'dead space'? Explain the difference between functional and anatomical dead space

Dead space is the volume of air within the lungs that does not take place in gaseous exchange.

Anatomical dead space –– This is the volume of the conducting airways that does not reach the alveoli. This includes air within the trachea and upper respiratory tract.

Alveolar dead space –– This is the volume of air contacting the alveoli without blood-flow in their adjacent pulmonary capillaries and hence not taking part in gaseous exchange.

Physiological dead space –– This is the anatomical dead space plus the alveolar dead space.

What is meant by minute ventilation?

This is the volume of air entering the lungs each minute. It is equal to the tidal volume multiplied by the respiratory rate (RR):

$$MV = TV \times RR$$

What is alveolar ventilation?

This is the volume of air entering the alveoli each minute. This takes into account the anatomical dead space:

$$\text{Alveolar Ventilation} = (TV - \text{anatomical dead space}) \times RR$$

Alveolar ventilation is a better measure of the level of ventilation. For example, a patient taking rapid, shallow breaths may have an adequate minute ventilation, but still be hypoxaemic, as an insufficient volume of inspired air is actually taking place in gaseous exchange.

What is Dalton's law of gases?

Dalton's law relates the concentration of a component gas within a mixture of gases to its partial pressure. It states that an individual gas (e.g., CO_2) within a mixture of gases in the alveolar space will be present in a concentration that is the same proportion as its partial pressure is of the total pressure.

What are the partial pressures of oxygen and carbon dioxide in inspired air?

$PO_2 = 21$ KPa; $PCO_2 = 0.03$ kPa

What are the partial pressures of oxygen and carbon dioxide in alveolar air?

$PO_2 = 14$ KPa; $PCO_2 = 5.3$ kPa

What are the normal partial pressures of oxygen and carbon dioxide in arterial blood?

$PO_2 = 13.3$ kPa; $PCO_2 = 5.3$ kPa.

Describe the alveolar gas equation and its relevance to clinical practice

This describes the inverse relationship between the arterial partial pressures of oxygen and carbon dioxide.

$$P_AO_2 = P_iO_2 - P_aCO_2/R$$

P_AO_2	Partial pressure of oxygen in arterial blood,
P_iO_2	Partial pressure of oxygen in inspired air,
P_ACO_2	Partial pressure of carbon dioxide in arterial blood,
P_aCO_2	Partial pressure of carbon dioxide in alveolar air,
R	Respiratory quotient.

Why is the partial pressure of carbon dioxide in the arterial blood virtually identical to that in alveolar air?

CO_2 is highly diffusible across the thin alveolar membrane. This is important in the derivation of the alveolar gas equation.

What is meant by lung compliance?

Compliance is the lungs ability to stretch, i.e., it is the change in volume per unit change in pressure. Overall lung compliance is approximately 200 ml/cmH$_2$O.

Which disease processes may influence lung compliance?

Emphysema and chronic obstructive pulmonary disease may *increase* pulmonary compliance as a result of loss of alveolar tissue and elasticity. Fibrosis, restrictive lung disease, pulmonary oedema and pulmonary venous congestion *reduce* compliance, as they reduce the lung's ability to stretch.

What is the role of surfactant in improving compliance in the normal lung?

Surfactant is produced by type II pneumocytes within the alveoli and is made up of lipid and protein components. It acts to decrease the surface tension within the alveolus present due to alveolar fluid. As a result, it prevents collapse of the alveolus on expiration and reduces the force required to overcome this surface tension, reducing the work of breathing. An additional role of surfactant is to reduce fluid transudation from the interstitium and prevent its accumulation within the alveolus.

Why are smaller alveoli more likely to collapse on lung deflation?

Laplace's law, when applied to the lung, states that pressure gradient across the alveolus (or transmural pressure, P) is equal to twice the wall tension (T) divided by the radius (r).

$$P = 2T/r$$

During expiration, r decreases. This means that a greater pressure is required to overcome the surface tension or the alveolus will collapse. It can therefore be seen that for smaller alveoli a larger transmural pressure is required to overcome the surface tension and prevent atelectasis during expiration.

What is elastance?

Elastance is a measure of the elastic recoil of the lung and it can be defined as 1/compliance. The main physiological mechanisms contributing to elastance are the alveolar surface tension and the elastin and collagen within the alveolar walls.

Chapter

4

Surgical approaches to the chest

What are the common approaches to the thoracic cavity?

Median sternotomy –– The patient is positioned supine on the operating table. A midline skin incision is made from the jugular notch to the xiphisternum. Using monopolar diathermy this is then extended through the subcutaneous fat, being careful to remain in the midline until the sternum is reached. Blunt dissection with a finger is then used to clear tissues below the xiphisternum and around the top of the manubrium. The interclavicular ligament is divided with diathermy and the xiphisternum is cut with McIndoes scissors. The sternal saw is then used to divide the bone and a retractor is placed to expose the anterior mediastinum.

Posterolateral thoracotomy –– The patient is positioned prone or in a lateral position dependent on the structures to be accessed. A long parascapular incision is made, running from a point midway between the medial scapular edge and the thoracic spine and following a curve that runs 2 cm below the inferior scapular angle, to the midpoint of the axilla.

Anterior thoracotomy –– The patient is positioned supine with elevation of the operative side using a sandbag. A submammary incision is made from the sternal edge anteriorly curving laterally along the intercostal space to the mid axillary line. The pectoralis fascia and serratus anterior are exposed. Pectoralis fascia and pectoralis major (medially) and the digitations of serratus anterior (laterally) are divided at the required level.

Posterior thoracotomy –– The line of the incision is similar to that of a posterolateral thoracotomy but starts more posteriorly. It crosses the inferior part of trapezius and posterior part of the latissimus dorsi and these are divided. This exposes the posterior border of the serratus anterior and the rhomboideus major. The attachments of the serratus are divided along with the rhomboid muscle and the scapula can be retracted. The incision is usually made in the fourth to fifth intercostal space but this is dependent on the structure to be accessed.

'Clamshell' incision (bilateral anterior sternotomy) –– The patient is positioned supine. Bilateral curvilinear submammary incisions are made at approximately the level of the sixth rib (the submammary fold). These extend from the anterior axillary line to meet at the midline. The pectoralis muscle is separated inferior and medially and lifted with the skin flap to expose the chest wall. The incision is then extended through the chest wall at the level of the fourth intercostal space. The sternum is divided at the same level with an oscillating saw. Care should be taken to identify the internal mammary vessels running along the anterior chest wall.

Thoraco-laparotomy –– The patient is positioned in the lateral decubitus position. The incision in the chest is the same as that of a posterolateral thoracotomy but it then continues anteriorly to cross the costal margin at the junction of the sixth and seventh ribs. The line runs for a further 5 cm into the abdominal wall and may continue into the abdomen either along the midline or as a paramedian incision dependent on the required access. Deep to the skin, the latissimus dorsi, serratus anterior and rectus sheath are divided with preservation of the rectus muscle by retraction towards the midline.

What structures are best accessed by each approach?

Median sternotomy –– Heart, pericardium, great vessels, thymus and both hemithoraces.

Anterior thoracotomy –– Lung and pericardial access, along with aortopulmonary window lymph nodes.

Posterior thoracotomy –– Lung and great vessels. Posterior thoracotomy is also used in some paediatric cardiac procedures, in particular PDA ligation.

Posterolateral thoracotomy –– Direct access to lung, tracheo-bronchial tree and mainstem bronchi. Posterolateral thoracotomy also provides access to aortopulmonary window (and is good for lymph node sampling).

Thoracolaparotomy –– Posterior mediastinal structures, in particular the descending thoracic aorta and distal oesophagus. Thoracolaparotomy can also be used to access the proximal stomach and colon. This approach may be used for re-do procedures and in older approaches to oesophagectomy and gastrectomy.

Clamshell incision –– Provides emergency access to the pericardium and heart, and provides simultaneous access to both pleural cavities.

How is the chest accessed during mediastinoscopy?

A 2 cm incision is made in the anterior neck two fingers breadth above the jugular notch. This allows access to the subcarinal lymph nodes for diagnosis and staging.

5

The mediastinum and diaphragm

Disorders of the thoracic aorta: aneurysms and dissection

Define what is meant by an aneurysm

True aneurysm –– This is a localized or diffuse dilatation of a blood vessel involving all three layers of the vessel wall. This dilatation is typically at least 50% greater than the normal size of the vessel and results from a weakness in the vessel wall itself.

False aneurysm –– This is caused by the formation of a haematoma following a leak from a vessel. Its wall is made up of fibrous connective tissue encapsulating the haematoma and is not the vessel wall itself. On clinical examination, this feels pulsatile and may have an overlying bruit.

How may aneurysms be classified?

1. True vs. false: see above,
2. According to shape: saccular or fusiform. (See Figure 5.1.)

Saccular –– This is a berry-like outpouching, which typically arises at the sites of arterial bifurcation. It is most commonly seen in the circle of Willis.

Fusiform –– This is an elongated, spindle shaped dilatation of a vessel – it is the type typically seen in atherosclerotic disease.

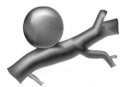

Saccular aneurysm

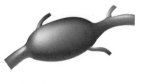

Fusiform aneurysm

Figure 5.1
Saccular and fusiform aneurysms.

What aetiological factors may lead to the development of aneurysms?

- Hypertension,
- Atherosclerosis,
- Infection (mycotic – often secondary to bacterial endocarditis),
- Trauma,
- Connective tissue disorders (Ehlers–Danlos, Marfan's syndrome),
- Cystic medial necrosis (post-stenotic).

Thoracic aortic dissection

What proportion of all thoracic aortic aneurysms are dissecting?

Approximately 25%. Distension of the arterial wall leads to a tear in the intima and the internal elastic lamina. This results in intramural haemorrhage and the development of a false lumen within the layers of the vessel wall. The underlying aetiology is usually atherosclerosis and hypertension, although less commonly aneurysms, may be caused by connective tissue disorders and cystic medial necrosis.

Who presents with aortic dissection?

Aortic dissection typically presents between ages 50 and 70. The male to female ratio is equal. The incidence is twice that of ruptured abdominal aortic aneurysm.

How is dissection of the thoracic aorta classified?

The Stanford classification

> **Type A**   dissection beginning just cranial to the right coronary artery.
>
> **Type B**   originates distal to the left subclavian artery.

The commonest site for an intimal tear is within 2–3 cm of the aortic valve. The second commonest site is just distal to the left subclavian artery. Type A may involve the aortic arch and the brachiocephalic trunk. It may also extend into the aortic root, leading to disruption of the aortic valve and the coronary ostia or coronary arteries. Type A aneurysms may also have a thoraco-abdominal extension (i.e., Type A + Type B).

The DeBakey classification (See Figure 5.2)

> **Type I (60%)**   Originates in the ascending aorta, propagates to the aortic arch and may extend beyond it distally,
>
> **Type II (10–15%)** Originates in and is confined to the ascending aorta,
>
> **Type III (25–30%)** Originates in the descending aorta, rarely extends proximally but extends distally.

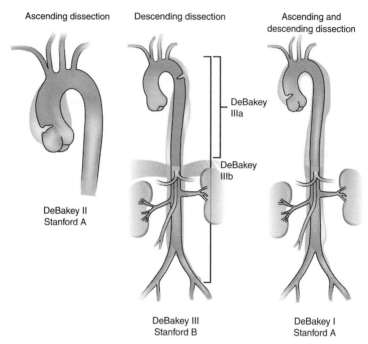

Ascending dissection

DeBakey II
Stanford A

Descending dissection

DeBakey
IIIa

DeBakey
IIIb

DeBakey III
Stanford B

Ascending and
descending dissection

DeBakey I
Stanford A

Figure 5.2 The DeBakey classification.

How does thoracic dissection typically present?

Symptoms –– Tearing chest pain radiating to the back, collapse.

Signs –– Reduced or absent peripheral pulses, unequal blood pressures L–R, early diastolic murmur of aortic regurgitation, pleural effusion, shock and pericardial tamponade.

The level of the dissection determines other presenting features. These may include: acute renal failure (renal arteries), acute limb ischaemia (iliac and femoral arteries), inferior myocardial infarction (right coronary artery), stroke (carotid arteries) and paraplegia (spinal arteries).

What investigations would you require?

Chest X-ray –– This may show widening of the mediastinum, pleural effusion, unfolding of the aorta with loss of the aortic knuckle and intimal calcium separated more than 6 mm from the vessel wall ('calcium sign').

Echocardiography –– Trans-oesophageal echocardiography has good sensitivity (98%) and specificity (97%). It may demonstrate an intimal flap and allows evaluation of the aortic valve and the coronary ostia. Visualization of the distal ascending aorta and descending aorta may, however, be poor.

CT scanning with IV contrast –– This allows visualization of the whole aorta and assessment of extent of the dissection. Its sensitivity and specificity is approximately 96–100%. In patients with renal failure, the use of contrast media is a relative contraindication. Other disadvantages include poor visualization of the intimal tear and inability to assess the competence of the aortic valve.

MRI –– This is the 'gold standard' investigation, with sensitivity and specificity of 98%: MRI scanning confers the advantages of CT without the need for contrast media, whilst also allowing assessment of the aortic valve.

What is the management of thoracic aortic dissection?

Medical management –– Treat associated hypertension. Aim to keep the mean arterial pressure 60–70 mmHg.

Surgical management –– Type A dissections are treated operatively. The aim of surgery is to excise the intimal tear, prevent progression of the dissection and excise the area likely to rupture. The approach is via median sternotomy, and the procedure requires cardiopulmonary bypass. The extent of the dissected portion of proximal aorta is excised, where possible sparing the aortic valve. A Dacron graft is then used to replace the excised length of aorta. Where the dissection extends into the aortic root and the valve is replaced, the coronary arteries must be re-anastamosed to the graft. Where the arch is involved, the same applies to the brachiocephalic, carotid and subclavian arteries. Operative mortality is between 25 and 30% dependent on the site and extent of the dissection. Without operation, mortality for type A dissections is 40% at 24 hours and 80% at 2 weeks.

Type B dissections are treated conservatively unless there is involvement of the renal or visceral arteries or imminent risk of rupture. Blood pressure must be very tightly controlled; this is usually with B-blockade and Nitroprusside. Surgery to type B dissections confers a high risk of paraplegia.

What are the contraindications to surgical intervention for thoracic aortic dissection?

Paraplegia (unlikely to resolve), and significant comorbidities contraindicating anaesthesia or surgery in general.

The diaphragm

Describe the structures penetrating the diaphragm and the corresponding vertebral levels at which these occur

    T8   Inferior vena cava, right phrenic nerve (note that the left phrenic nerve passes separately and pierces the muscular portion of the diaphragm),

    T10   Oesophagus, vagus nerve,

    T12   Abdominal aorta, azygous vein, thoracic duct.

Which other structures pierce or cross the diaphragm?

- The greater, lesser and least splanchnic nerves pierce the crura of the diaphragm.
- The sympathetic chain passes behind the medial arcuate ligament.

Diaphragmatic herniae: pathophysiology and treatment

What structures are involved in the embryological development of the diaphragm?

The septum transversum (becomes the central tendon), the dorsal oesophageal mesentery and the pleuroperitoneal membranes. The crura of the diaphragm are derived from foregut mesenchyme.

What are the common sites for congenital diaphragmatic herniae?

The foramen of Morgagni (through the anterior steno-costal portion of the diaphragm) and the foramen of Bochdalek (located postero-laterally, usually on the left). Herniation through the foramen on Morgagni is usually small and clinically unimportant. Herniation through the foramen of Bochdalek is usually large and presents with respiratory distress soon after birth, requiring urgent surgical intervention.

Briefly outline the clinical presentation of a traumatic diaphragmatic hernia

These typically present after either blunt crush injury to the upper abdomen or thorax or after direct penetrating injury. The patient is usually unwell and may have multiple other traumatic injuries. Chest radiography may show herniation of the stomach (gastric bubble) into the thoracic cavity or loss of the diaphragmatic contour on one side. The left side is more commonly injured than the right, which is protected by the liver. Traumatic diaphragmatic herniae require urgent surgical repair and other thoracic or abdominal injury must also be ruled out by relevant investigations or exploration.

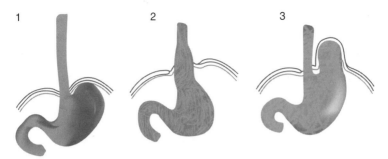

Figure 5.3 Classification of hiatus herniae: (1) no hernia, (2) sliding hernia, (3) rolling hernia.

Hiatus herniae: pathophysiology and treatment

What is meant by a hiatus hernia and how may they be classified?

A hiatus hernia is the protrusion of a portion of the stomach through the diaphragmatic hiatus (see Figure 5.3). Hiatus herniae may be either sliding (90%) or rolling (10%). Hiatus herniae are generally more common in women than in men.

What is the difference between a sliding and rolling hiatus hernia?

Sliding –– The gastro-oesophageal junction slides through the oesophageal hiatus. There is disruption of the lower oesophageal sphincter (LOS) and a predisposition to reflux and Barrett's oesophagus.

Rolling –– A portion of the fundus of the stomach (covered with peritoneum) herniates anteriorly through the oesophageal hiatus alongside the LOS but the cardia remains in the abdominal cavity. There are not typically symptoms of reflux as the LOS mechanism is intact.

Which investigations may be used to confirm the diagnosis?

It is important to confirm the diagnosis by means of upper GI endoscopy (biopsy to show oesophagitis or Barrett's oesophagus) and 24 h lower oesophageal pH recording.

List the key points in the management of hiatus hernia

The majority of hiatus herniae are incidental findings on endoscopy and if asymptomatic require no formal management. In symptomatic patients, the following management strategies may be used:

Lifestyle modification

- Weight loss,
- Alcohol avoidance,

- Smoking cessation,
- Avoiding large meals or eating late at night,
- Elevating the head of the bed during sleep.

Medical

Antacids	Both aluminium- and magnesium-containing salts are used as acid-neutralizing agents and relieve the symptoms of dyspepsia. Examples include: aluminium hydroxide, magnesium carbonate, magnesium hydroxide and magnesium trisilicate. Magnesium salts may have a laxative effect, whereas aluminium salts may be constipating, therefore combination therapy may be used to alleviate these colonic side effects.
Bismuth salts and Sucralfate	Improve mucosal repair. Sucralfate may also partially reduce acid secretion and suppress *Helicobacter pylori* infection.
Prostaglandin analogues (e.g., misoprostol)	May increase mucosal resistance and exert a weak acid suppressive effect
Histamine receptor (H_2) antagonists (e.g., Ranitidine, Cimetidine)	Useful in mild oesophagitis, H_2 antagonists inhibit histamine binding to H_2 receptors on the parietal cell and as a result reduce acid secretion.
Proton pump inhibitors (PPIs) (e.g., Omeprazole, Lansoprazole)	Inhibit H^+ ion secretion by the parietal cell by irreversibly inhibiting the H^+/K^+ ATPase membrane transporter.

Surgical

Nissen's fundoplication (most common)	Less commonly used approaches include the Belsey Mark IV (fundoplication through a thoracotomy) and Hill gastropexy (the cardia of the stomach is anchored to the pre-aortic fascia).

What are the indications for surgical intervention?

The indications for anti-reflux surgery are largely relative rather than absolute and include:

1. Complications associated with reflux disease, e.g., stricture, bleeding and ulceration or pulmonary complications (aspiration, hoarseness, recurrent chest infections),

2. Persistent regurgitation despite medical management,
3. Patient choice.

Briefly describe the operative technique involved in Nissen's fundoplication

Nissen's fundoplication, whilst traditionally performed by an open technique, is now most almost always performed laparoscopically.

- The patient is positioned supine; the primary surgeon may either stand to the side of the patient or between the legs.
- A 10 mm port is inserted in the supraumbilical position and pneumoperitoneum is established. Four further 5 mm ports are inserted: two in the right and two in the left hypochondrium.
- The liver retractor is inserted into the first right hypochondrial port to allow the left lobe of the liver to be retracted, exposing the stomach and gastro-oesophageal junction. The assistant then retracts the stomach caudally to allow dissection of the right crus of the diaphragm.
- The left crus of the diaphragm is now dissected by division of the phreno-oesophageal ligament anteriorly. Care must be taken not to injure the anterior vagus nerve during the dissection.
- The distal 3–4 cm of oesophagus is mobilized, taking care to avoid damage to the posterior vagus nerve on dissection around the posterior oesophagus. A Penrose drain may be passed around the oesophagus to allow it to be retracted anteriorly to facilitate this dissection.
- The fundus of the stomach is now mobilized and passed through the window that has been created posterior to the oesophagus. This creates the fundal wrap (this should be 'short and floppy' and should not be under tension).
- At this point, the right and left crura are approximated posterior to the oesophagus to recreate the oesophageal hiatus.
- The fundal wrap is then secured with two or three interrupted non-absorbable sutures, ensuring muscular bites from the fundus and partial thickness from the oesophagus.
- Irrigation of the operative field is performed and haemostasis is ensured prior to port site closure.

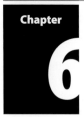

Chapter 6

The breast: benign and malignant disease

What are the four most common causes of a breast lump?

- Breast carcinoma,
- Fibroadenoma,
- Simple breast cyst,
- Localized anomaly of breast development and involution (ANDI).

Less common causes include: fat necrosis (where there is a history of trauma), other breast cysts (galactocele, cystadenoma, retention cyst of gland of Montgomery), breast abscess (clinical signs of infection) and lipoma.

How does the differential diagnosis of a breast mass vary with age?

A large proportion of breast lumps are found to be benign lesions; however, malignancy becomes more prevalent with increasing age. In adolescence and early adulthood, fibroadenomas and other benign lesions make up the majority of breast lumps. By the age of 55 years, malignancy accounts for up to 85% of all breast lumps. Cystic breast disease is most prevalent in patients aged 40–55 years (accounting for approximately 25% of breast lumps), although it should be noted that cancer is still more common in this age group.

Benign disease
What is a fibroadenoma?

Fibroadenomas are benign breast lesions arising from the epithelium and stromal cells of the duct lobule. They are well defined, freely mobile, have a smooth edge, and are usually less than 5 cm in diameter (>5 cm is classified as a giant fibroadenoma). Fibroadenomas are most commonly found in the upper, outer quadrant and may be multiple or bilateral (approximately 10–15%).

What is the key histological feature of fibroadenoma?

Proliferation of both glandular and stromal cellular elements is observed.

At what age do fibroadenomas most commonly occur?

At 15–30 years. Fibroadenomas are hormonally dependent lesions, which involute after the menopause.

What are the common clinical features of a breast cyst?

Breast cysts most commonly occur in women aged 40–55 years and may be associated with a history of hormone replacement therapy. Breast cysts typically present as either single or multiple smooth, well-defined, fluctuant breast lumps, which may be painful.

Which features of a breast mass are suspicious of malignancy?

Appearance –– Overlying skin tethering, irregularity, involvement of the nipple (Paget's disease of the nipple is associated with underlying intraductal carcinoma in 50% of cases), bloody discharge from nipple, peu d'orange, absence of signs of infection (e.g., cellulitis and skin erythema).

Feel –– Hard, poorly defined, irregular, solid mass which is non-tender and without fluctuance (suggestive of an abscess).

Local and metastatic invasion –– Fixation to the underlying muscle, axillary lymphadenopathy, symptoms and signs of metastatic disease (e.g., bone pain and shortness of breath).

Breast cancer: diagnosis, investigation and management

What is the incidence of breast cancer in the UK?

The age-standardized incidence rate is 123.9 per 100 000 women and 65.2 per 100 000 of men and women (Cancer research UK, 2008 data). The lifetime risk of breast cancer is one in eight for all UK women. It is the commonest cancer in the UK (excluding non-melanoma skin cancer).

Which risk factors are associated with breast cancer?

Age –– The risk of breast cancer is significantly higher in women older than 50 years.

Family history –– The lifetime risk is increased to one in four in patients with a premenopausal first-degree relative with confirmed breast cancer. This risk is approximately one in seven where the first-degree relative was postmenopausal at the time of diagnosis.

Genetics –– BRCA-1 (chromosome 17) and BRCA-2 (chromosome 13) are autosomal dominant genes, accounting for 2–3% of all breast cancers. BRCA gene mutations confer a 45–65% risk of developing breast cancer by age 70 years.

Hormonal
- Increased risk:
  - Early menarche and late menopause,
  - Nulliparity women and later age at first pregnancy,
  - Hormone replacement therapy (HRT),
- Potentially reduced risk:
  - Breastfeeding.

Environmental and lifestyle –– Exposure to ionizing radiation, obesity and alcohol consumption may increase risk. Long-term use of non-steroidal anti-inflammatory drugs may reduce the risk of breast cancer.

Benign breast disease –– Benign breast disease with atypical hyperplasia or proliferative breast disease without atypica increases the relative risk of breast cancer development.

History –– Previous breast cancer or carcinoma *in situ*.

What are the key histological subtypes of breast cancer and what are their key features?

Ductal carcinoma in situ (DCIS) –– This is the most common histological subtype detected on mammograms, appearing as a branching microcalcification. Histologically, it is characterized by malignant proliferation of epithelial cells, bounded by the ductal basement membrane. Further classification of DCIS may then be according to the cellular architecture: solid, cribriform, papillary and micropapillary; the tumour grade: high, intermediate, and low; and whether comedo necrosis is present. Patients with DCIS are at increased risk of developing invasive carcinoma. Oestrogen receptor (ER) positivity may be linked with a decreased risk of recurrence of DCIS, whereas HER-2 (human epidermal growth factor-2) positivity has been linked to an increased risk of recurrence.

Invasive ductal carcinoma (IDC) –– This accounts for approximately 75% of all breast cancers. The majority of invasive ductal carcinomas are of 'no special subtype' (NOS), although other less common subtypes include medullary, mucinous, cribriform, tubular and papillary. Clinically, IDC usually presents as a firm, irregular palpable mass and features of lymphatic invasion (peu d'orange, axillary node involvement) and local inflammation (Paget's disease of the nipple) may be present. Histologically, infiltration of clusters of malignant cells is seen within a dense, fibrous stroma.

Lobular carcinoma in situ (LCIS) -- Lobular carcinoma *in situ* is not usually detectable on mammograms and lacks any specific clinical features. Histologically, it is characterized by proliferation of terminal duct-lobular unit cells. The lobular units become filled and distorted with tumour cells. Classically LCIS is EGFR-1 and HER-2 negative but ER and PR (progesterone receptor) positive. The cumulative risk for invasive carcinoma is estimated at 18% (ipsilateral) and 14% (contralateral), of which 40% are lobular and 60% are ductal tumours.[1]

Invasive lobular carcinoma -- This accounts for approximately 8–14% of all invasive breast cancers and its incidence is increasing. Invasive lobular carcinoma more frequently presents as multifocal, bilateral or diffuse lesions. Histologically it is characterized by small, round cells with scanty cytoplasm, which form a linear 'rosary' pattern. Invasive lobular carcinoma does not form well-circumscribed masses and generally does not distort surrounding structures in the early stages, often precluding diagnosis by fine needle aspiration.

How is a breast mass investigated?

Triple test Examination, ultrasound and cytology (fine needle aspiration or core biopsy).

This is the 'gold standard' for investigation and diagnosis of breast masses. In patients up to 40 years old, ultrasound is used to define the lesion and characterize any cystic, solid or calcific components. Mammography is not used in this age group, as the image quality is poor due to the dense fibro-glandular nature of the breast tissue. In patients older than 40 years, mammography replaces ultrasound in the triple assessment. The sensitivity of mammography varies with age but is overall estimated at approximately 85% in women over 50. It may, however be as low as 62% in women 40–49 years old (International Agency for Research on Cancer).

Which further investigations may be performed where there is confirmed evidence of malignancy?

MRI -- Routine breast MRI is not recommended where invasive cancer or ductal carcinoma *in situ* is confirmed. However, it should be offered in patients with invasive cancer where there is a discrepancy over the extent of disease on triple assessment, if accurate mammographic assessment is not possible or where breast-conserving surgery is being considered for invasive lobular cancer (*NICE Guidance, CG80*).

---

[1] Data from M. Hussain and G. H. Cunnick (2011). Management of lobular carcinoma *in-situ* and atypical lobular hyperplasia of the breast – a review. *EJSO*, **37**(4):279–89.

Axillary ultrasound – Is used where there is confirmed evidence of early invasive cancer to assess for local lymph node abnormality. Where abnormal lymph nodes are identified, it is recommended that ultrasound-guided biopsy be performed prior to surgery.

PET CT – The role of PET is largely in the detection of multifocal disease, assessment of metastatic disease, and where recurrence is suspected.

Nuclear scanning, e.g., ^{99m}Tc: – This may be used in assessing metastatic disease or the response to treatment.

What is the role of breast cancer screening in the UK?

The NHS national breast cancer screening programme was set up in 1988 and offers screening every three years to all women age 50–70 years. Two-view mammography is now taken at every screen and each film is read by two independent assessors. The results are sent to the patient's GP. Where there is suspicion of an abnormality, the patient is recalled for completion of a formal triple assessment. There is currently a move to extend this age range from 47–73 years, which should be completely phased in by 2012.

How is breast cancer staged?

Staging is according to the TNM system:

Primary tumour

Tis Carcinoma *in situ*. Divided into: T_{DCIS} – ductal carcinoma *in situ*; T_{LCIS} – lobular carcinoma *in situ*; T_{Paget} – Paget's disease of the nipple not associated with invasive carcinoma DCIS or LCIS,

T1 $\leq$20 mm in greatest diameter. Divided into T1mi – $\leq$1 mm; T1a – >1 mm but $\leq$5 mm; T1b – >5 mm but $\leq$10 mm; T1c – >10 mm but $\leq$20 mm,

T2 Tumour size >20 mm but $\leq$50 mm in greatest diameter,

T3 Tumour size >50 mm in greatest diameter,

T4 Tumour of any size, which directly invades the chest wall or surrounding skin. Divided into: T4a – invasion into the chest wall (although invasion into the pectoralis muscle alone does not qualify as a T4 lesion); T4b – ulceration, surrounding skin oedema (peu d'orange) or ipsilateral satellite nodules (isolated dermal invasion does not qualify for T4b); T4c – both T4a and T4b; T4c – inflammatory carcinoma.

Lymph nodes

N0 No lymph node involvement,

N1 Clinically detectable, mobile level I or II axillary nodes on the ipsilateral side as the lesion,

N2   Immobile, fixed ipsilateral axillary lymph nodes (N2a) or clinically detectable ipsilateral internal mammary node metastases, without axillary node involvement (N2b),

N3   N3a – infraclavicular lymph node involvement; N3b – both internal mammary and axillary lymph node involvement; N3c – supraclavicular lymph node involvement.

Distant metastases

M0   No distant metastases,

cM0 (i+)   No clinically detectable metastases, but tumour cells (<0.2mm) detectable in blood, bone marrow or non-nodal tissue (without clinical signs of metastases),

M1   Clinically detectable distant metastases or histologically proven metastases >0.2mm diameter.

Which hormonal receptors affect the course of tumour progression and may be exploited in cancer treatment?

ER/PR –– ER- and PR- (progesterone receptor) positive tumours usually have a more indolent course and are responsive to hormonal therapy.

HER-2 –– Tumours displaying HER-2 overexpression are usually of a more aggressive phenotype and confer a worse prognosis without specific hormonal therapy.

Briefly describe the non-surgical management of breast carcinoma

Radiotherapy –– All patients with intermediate or high-risk early invasive carcinoma should be offered adjuvant breast radiotherapy (usually a five-week course) following wide local excision (WLE) or mastectomy to reduce the risk of recurrence (provided there is no absolute contraindication). Breast radiotherapy is also recommended following breast-conserving surgery for DCIS. Nodal radiotherapy is offered in lymph-node-positive disease. Side effects of radiotherapy include skin desquamation, erythema and permanent skin discoloration, lymphoedema, arm weakness and, more rarely, brachial plexopathy and pulmonary fibrosis.

Chemotherapy –– Adjuvant chemotherapy in early-stage breast cancer may reduce the risk of both disease recurrence and death. It is most effective in premenopausal women. Combination chemotherapy involves anthracycline-based regimens (cyclophosphamide, doxorubicin), with docetaxyl added in lymph-node-positive disease. As with adjuvant radiotherapy, it is recommended that adjuvant chemotherapy be commenced within one month of surgery. Neo-adjuvant chemotherapy may be beneficial in large tumours or inflammatory cancers.

Hormonal therapy –– Categories of hormonal therapy include:

1. *Selective oestrogen receptor modulators (SERMs) – Tamoxifen and Raloxifine.* Tamoxifen may be used to reduce the risk of cancer recurrence or as prophylaxis in women at higher risk of breast cancer development. It is typically given as 20 mg/day for a five-year course.

2. *Aromatase inhibitors (e.g., anastrazole, lestrazole).* These work by reducing systemic oestrogen levels. Currently, aromatase inhibitors are recommended as first-line adjuvant therapy in postmenopausal women with non-low-risk ER positive tumours.

Monoclonal antibody therapy –– *Trastuzumab (Herceptin)* is a monoclonal antibody, which binds to HER-2 causing an antibody-mediated destruction of cells overexpressing HER-2.

Briefly describe the principles of the surgical treatment of breast cancer

Surgery is commonly the first definitive treatment in patients with DCIS and invasive carcinoma.

Wide local excision (WLE) –– This is most commonly indicated in patients with DCIS and unifocal early invasive cancer. Local excision may also potentially be possible in Paget's disease of the nipple. A minimum margin of 2 mm is recommended in WLE for DCIS although margins of up to 1 cm have been advocated in invasive carcinoma. Where histology shows incomplete clearance, re-excision of margins should be performed. Conservation of breast tissue reduces the side effects of radical excision; however, it may increase the need for re-intervention to achieve adequate excision margins and be associated with higher rates of disease recurrence.

Mastectomy –– The degree of tissue removed during mastectomy varies according to clinical indication. A *simple mastectomy* involves excision of the entire breast tissue, sparing the axillary contents. In a *modified ('Patey') radical mastectomy* the breast tissue, pectoralis minor and axillary contents are excised. The *'Halstead' radical mastectomy* is now rarely performed, except where there is involvement of the pectoral muscles and chest wall. This procedure involves excision of the entire breast tissue, pectoralis major and minor and the axillary contents. It leads to significant cosmetic disfigurement and surgical side effects. The indications for mastectomy include multifocal disease, large tumours relative to breast size and recurrence following local re-excision. Prophylactic mastectomy may also be offered in patients testing positive for BRCA 1 and 2 mutations.

The axilla

Sentinel node biopsy   Sentinel node biopsy is the recommended technique for axillary staging in patients with early tumours with ultrasound or FNA-negative axillary nodes. The sentinel node is the first node to receive lymphatic drainage from the tumour site and is therefore the first to be infiltrated by tumour cells. The technique involves a series of peri-tumour injections of either blue dye or radioisotope followed by direct visualization or radio-uptake scanning of the axilla to determine the sentinel node. This node is then excised and examined histologically for the presence of metastases. Where metastatic disease is present, formal excision of this group of nodes is performed, thereby minimizing necessary axillary clearance. It is notable that sentinel node biopsy is not used in palpable lymph node metastases, as infiltration of these nodes with tumour cells blocks uptake of the tracer, leading to false negatives.

Axillary clearance   Complete axillary clearance involves excision of all lymph nodes below the axillary vein (i.e., Level I, II and III nodes). The dissection extends anteriorly to the pectoralis muscles, medially to the chest wall, laterally to the axillary skin and posteriorly to the latissimus dorsi, teres major and subscapularis. Care must be taken to avoid injury to the intercostobrachial nerve and smaller cutaneous branches to the axillary skin.

How are the axillary nodes classified?

Level I   Inferolateral to pectoralis minor,

Level II   Posterior to pectoralis minor,

Level III   Superomedial to pectoralis minor.

Which reconstructive options are available after mastectomy?

Reconstruction may be performed either immediately following resection (single procedure) or as a staged procedure. Where immediate reconstruction is not contraindicated by the need for adjuvant therapy or patient comorbidities, it should be discussed with the patient prior to surgery. Several approaches to reconstruction exist: common approaches to reconstruction include implant reconstruction, TRAM (transverse rectus abdominis muscle) flap, DIEP (deep inferior epigastric perforator) flap and latissimus dorsi flap. Other examples include gracilis and gluteal myocutaneous flaps.

Implant reconstruction -- This may be part of a single or two-stage procedure. In patients with small breasts where sufficient skin can be preserved, immediate reconstruction with a silicone or saline implant may be possible. Where there is insufficient skin to prevent excess tension, a tissue expander may be placed which is gradually inflated, creating space for a permanent implant. The expander is then removed and the implant inserted in a second procedure. Either saline or silicone implants may be used, most commonly placed subpectorally.

Pedicled TRAM flap -- A transverse abdominal incision is made and a myocutaneous flap involving abdominal skin, underlying fat and the rectus muscle is raised. This is then tunnelled between the abdomen and anterior chest to reconstruct the breast. The blood supply to the flap is the deep superior epigastric artery supplying the rectus muscle, feeding the myocutaneous perforator vessels, which supply the skin.

'Free' TRAM flap -- This technique involves mobilization of the lower rectus muscle and attached inferior epigastric vessels. This flap is then lifted free and transposed into the defect, where a vascular anastomosis with the thoracodorsal or internal mammary vessels is performed.

DIEP flap -- This technique involves raising a flap of skin and underlying fat over one of the deep epigastric perforator vessels. Its benefits over the TRAM flap include sparing the rectus muscle and minimizing the donor site defect. The DIEP flap is, however, technically more demanding and may result in higher rates of venous congestion and flap necrosis.

Latissimus dorsi flap -- This technique mobilizes a myocutaneous flap including an island of skin and the ipsilateral latissimus dorsi muscle. The flap is then tunnelled through the axilla to the anterior chest wall to create the reconstruction.

What are the complications of mastectomy?

Immediate -- Bleeding and haematoma formation.

Early -- Infection, haematoma, seroma, numbness and paraesthesiae over breast, skin flap necrosis, excess skin at the corners of wide skin excision ('dog ears'), thoracodorsal and long thoracic nerve injury (weakness of latissimus dorsi and serratus anterior respectively), breast oedema.

Late -- Tumour recurrence.

What are the complications of axillary clearance?

Immediate -- Bleeding and haematoma formation

Early -- Infection, haematoma, seroma, intercostobrachial nerve injury, reduced upper limb mobility.

Late -- Lymphoedema and tumour recurrence.

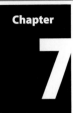

Chapter **Applied surgical anatomy**

7

Which two fascial layers lie in the subcutaneous tissue beneath the anterior abdominal wall?

Camper's fascia –– Most superficial, thin fatty layer of subcutaneous fascia.

Scarpa's fascia –– Strong membranous layer of fascia lying beneath Camper's fascia. Scarpa's fascia also continues over the scrotum and penis as the superficial perineal fascia and attaches to the fascia lata of the thigh just below the inguinal ligament.

Describe the four main muscles of the anterior abdominal wall, their origins and insertions

External oblique

Origin	Fifth–twelfth ribs.
Insertion	The lower fibres insert onto the anterior half of the lilac crest. The upper fibres form an aponeurosis, which extends medially to the linea alba. The lower border of the external oblique aponeurosis forms the inguinal ligament.
Direction of fibres	Inferoanterior.

Internal oblique

Origin	Lumbosacral fascia, anterior two-thirds of the iliac crest and lateral two-thirds of the inguinal ligament.
Insertion	The linea alba, xiphoid process and inferior border of the tenth to twelfth ribs.
Direction of fibres	Superomedial.

Note: The lower border of the internal oblique arches over the spermatic cord forming the external ring (consequently, laterally the fibres of the internal oblique are anterior to the cord but medially they pass posterior to the cord).

Transversus abdominis

Origin	Lateral third of the inguinal ligament, the anterior two-thirds of the iliac crest, the lumbar fascia, the twelfth rib and the inner part of the lower six costal cartilages.
Insertion	The lower fibres insert onto the pubic crest and the pectineal line, forming the conjoint tendon. The upper fibres insert into the linea alba.

Rectus abdominis

Origin	The medial head arises from the pubic symphysis, lateral head from the pubic crest.
Insertion	The front of the fifth to seventh costal cartilages.

Which structure makes up the semilunar line?

The splitting of the internal oblique aponeurosis down the lateral border of the rectus muscle.

Which two layers of the abdominal wall form the conjoint tendon? What is its insertion?

The internal oblique and transversus abdominis form the conjoint tendon. Its insertion is the pubic crest and pectineal line.

What or where is the arcuate line (semicircular line of Douglas)?

Midway between the umbilicus and the pubic symphysis. Here, the posterior layer of the internal oblique ends and both layers pass anterior to the rectus muscle. The aponeurosis of transversus abdominis also passes posterior to the recti inferior to this line.

Which structures lie within the rectus sheath?

The lower sixth intercostal nerves (T7–T11) and the superior and inferior epigastric vessels.

What are the boundaries of the Lumbar triangle of Petit and what is the significance of this region?

This is the site of the rare inferior lumbar hernia (of Petit).

Floor	Internal oblique,
Posteriorly	Anterior border of latissimus dorsi,
Inferiorly	Iliac crest.

The peritoneal cavity

Which structures make up the anterior and posterior borders of the lesser sac?

Anterior wall –– The peritoneum covering the lesser omentum, the posterior wall of the stomach and the anterior two layers of the greater omentum.

Posterior wall –– The posterior two layers of the greater omentum, the anterior surface of the transverse mesocolon and the transverse colon. Above the attachment of the transverse mesocolon, the posterior wall of the lesser sac is formed by the peritoneum covering the diaphragm, pancreas, left kidney and adrenal, abdominal aorta and coeliac artery.

Name the opening into the lesser sac

Epiploic foramen or foramen of Winslow.

What are the borders of this foramen?

Posteriorly –– Inferior vena cava (IVC).

Anteriorly –– Free border of the lesser omentum – containing the portal vein (posterior), hepatic artery (left anterior) and common bile duct (right anterior).

Superiorly –– Caudate process of the liver.

Inferiorly –– First part of the duodenum.

How may you approach the lesser sac surgically?

The commonest method is by lifting the greater omentum and incising the avascular plane between the omentum and the transverse colon.

The foregut

What is the embryological origin of the alimentary canal?

The gut is derived from endoderm. In the fourth week, the embryo folds both ventrally and laterally. The cranial fold incorporates part of the yolk sac into the embryo, creating the primordial foregut. In a similar fashion, the caudal and lateral folds create the primordial hindgut and midgut, respectively. After folding, the originally wide connection between the gut tube and the yolk sac is reduced to the narrow 'yolk stalk' or vitelline duct. (Clinical relevance: the Meckel's diverticulum is the vestigial remnant of the vitelline duct.)

Which vessel supplies the foregut, what are its branches and at which vertebral level does it arise?

The coeliac trunk, arising at the level of T12, with three branches.

1. Left gastric artery (supplies lower third of oesophagus and stomach along lesser curve),
2. Splenic artery (supplies pancreas and spleen),
3. Common hepatic arteries (supplies stomach, pancreas and liver).

What is the course of the common hepatic artery?

The common hepatic artery runs along the upper border of the pancreas to the free edge of the lesser omentum, where it lies anterior to the portal vein and to the left of the CBD. It divides into the *left and right hepatic* arteries at the *porta hepatis*.

Name the branches of the splenic artery

1. Short gastric arteries (usually six), running in the gastrosplenic ligament,
2. Left gastro-epiploic artery, running in the greater omentum along the greater curve of the stomach,
3. Posterior gastric artery, supplying the stomach.

Name the branches of the common hepatic artery

1. Right gastric: runs along the lesser curve of the stomach where it anastamoses with the left gastric artery.
2. Gastroduodenal: passes behind the first part of the duodenum and divides into the right gastro-epiploic and superior pancreaticoduodenal arteries.

Which of these vessels make up the blood supply to the stomach?

Origin	Coeliac trunk,
Lesser curve	Left gastric, right gastric,
Fundus and upper left part of greater curve	Short gastrics (six),
Remainder of greater curve	Right and left gastro-epiploic arteries.

Where would you find the transpyloric plane of Addison?

Midway between the xiphisternum and the umbilicus.

Which structures lie in this plane?

1. The body of L1,
2. The fundus of the gallbladder,
3. The pylorus of the stomach,
4. The duodeno-jejunal junction,
5. The origin of the superior mesenteric artery,
6. The formation of the portal vein from the superior mesenteric and splenic veins,

7. The hilum of the spleen,
8. The hilum of both kidneys,
9. The neck of the pancreas,
10. The origin of the transverse mesocolon,
11. The termination of the spinal cord.

Which vessels make up the portal vein and where does it form?

The portal vein forms from the superior mesenteric and splenic veins. The inferior mesenteric vein joins the splenic vein in front of the left crus of the diaphragm prior to the formation of the portal vein.

Site –– The portal vein is formed behind the head of the pancreas and in front of the IVC.

List five sites of porto-systemic anastamoses

1. Lower part of the oesophagus (approx T8) – azygous system in upper part (systemic), left gastric lower part (portal);
2. Upper third of the anal canal – upper third of the superior rectal and IMV (portal), lower two-thirds of the middle and inferior rectal to internal iliac veins (systemic);
3. Bare area of the liver – hepatic veins drain directly to IVC (systemic), portal venous channels in the liver (portal);
4. Peri-umbilical region – paraumbilical veins in the ligamentum teres drain to the portal vein (portal), subcutaneous venous network drains to great saphenous and lateral thoracic veins (systemic);
5. Retroperitoneum – drainage of ascending and descending colon (portal), posterior abdominal wall (systemic).

The midgut

Which point marks the end of the foregut and beginning of the midgut?

The entrance of the bile duct into the duodenum.

Which artery forms the blood supply to the midgut and at which vertebral level does it arise?

Superior mesenteric artery (SMA); L1.

List the key branches of the SMA

Inferior pancreaticoduodenal artery –– Runs between the duodenum and head of the pancreas and anastamoses with the superior pancreaticoduodenal artery.

Jejunal and ileal branches –– Form the mesenteric arcades.

Ileocolic artery –– Descends to the RIF and supplies the terminal ileum, caecum, appendix (via appendicular artery) and part of the ascending colon.

R colic artery –– Supplies the right colon up to the hepatic flexure.

Middle colic artery –– Supplies the transverse colon up to the splenic flexure: here it anastamoses with the L colic artery, a branch of the inferior mesenteric artery (IMA).

At its origin, the middle colic lies to the right of the midline and as such leaves an avascular area in the transverse mesocolon, often known as the watershed area.

Briefly describe the nervous supply to the gut

There are three key extrinsic plexi: coeliac, para-aortic and inferior hypogastric plexi.

Two intrinsic plexi are found within the wall of the gut, these receive excitatory preganglionic parasympathetic and inhibitory postganglionic sympathetic fibres:

- Myenteric (Auerbach's) plexus, between the muscle layers,
- Submucosal (Meissener's) plexus, in the submucosal layer.

Which parts of the colon are supported by mesentery?

Transverse and sigmoid colon. The ascending and descending colon are devoid of peritoneum posteriorly and adhere to the posterior abdominal wall. In 20% of the population, however, the descending colon also has an associated mesentery.

The hindgut

What is the marginal artery of Drummond and what does it supply?

This vessel forms the junction between the SMA and IMA. From here, shorter vessels run to supply the gut wall. Its area of relative deficiency is between the middle and left colic vessels. This area is supplied by the inner arterial arc of Riolan between the ascending branch of the left colic artery and the trunk of the middle colic.

What are the peritoneal relations to the rectum?

Upper third	Covered by peritoneum anteriorly and laterally,
Middle third	Covered by peritoneum anteriorly,
Lower third	Lies below the level of the peritoneal reflection.

Where is the pouch of Douglas?

The pouch of Douglas (or rectouterine or rectovesical pouch) is the cavity formed by the peritoneal reflection between the rectum and the bladder in the male or the posterior wall of the uterus in the female.

What and where is Denonviller's fascia?

This is the fascia separating the prostate and bladder base from the rectum. It connects the floor of the pouch of Douglas to the apex of the prostate and is formed from a condensation of the mesorectal fascia forming the rectogenital septum. It is divided; the layer coating the rectum is usually removed in oncological resections of the rectum.

What is the blood supply to the rectum?

The superior rectal, middle rectal, inferior rectal and median sacral arteries.

The IMA becomes the superior rectal vessel as it runs in the rectal mesentery and crosses the pelvic brim. The median sacral vessels also enter the mesorectum posteriorly at the anorectal junction, and they must be carefully divided during TME dissection, to avoid inadvertent bleeding.

What is the lymphatic drainage of the rectum?

The rectum drains to the epicolic and para-rectal nodes in the mesorectum. This then follows the IMA to the pre-aortic nodes. Mesorectal node involvement is an important consideration in excisions for rectal cancer.

The abdominal aorta

List the vertebral levels corresponding to the origins of the coeliac axis, SMA, IMA, renal arteries, adrenal arteries and gonadal arteries

Coeliac axis	T12,
SMA	L1,
IMA	L3,
Renal arteries	L2,
Adrenal arteries	T12,
Gonadal arteries	L2–L3.

At which level does the abdominal aorta bifurcate?

L4 (into common iliac vessels).

What are the branches of the internal iliac artery?

Posterior division –– Ileolumbar, lateral sacral and superior gluteal.

Anterior division –– Superior vesical, inferior vesical, middle rectal, vaginal, uterine, obturator, internal pudendal and inferior gluteal.

How is the spread of pelvic metastases to the lumbar vertebrae explained by the anatomy of the pelvic venous system?

The lateral sacral veins allow communication of the internal iliac vein with the vertebral venous plexuses. A sudden increase in intra-abdominal pressure may produce a venous pressure greater than the IVC can accommodate and so blood may be driven back up into the vertebral venous plexuses to the posterior intercostals and finally into the azygous system and SVC.

It is, however, notable that the usual mode of spread of pelvic tumours to the sacrum is via direct invasion.

The anus

Which nerves innervate the internal anal sphincter?

Sympathetic fibres of the inferior hypogastric plexus are motor to the internal sphincter.

What is the length of the anal canal?

4 cm (although may be shorter in women).

Describe the characteristics of the internal anal sphincter

The internal anal sphincter is visceral smooth muscle. It is a downward continuation of the inner circular muscle of the rectum, and is found to extend three-quarters of the length of the anal canal.

Describe the characteristics of the external anal sphincter

The external anal sphincter is skeletal muscle and is continuous with levator ani. It comprises three components: subcutaneous, superficial and deep. Its nerve supply arises from the inferior haemorrhoidal branch of the pudendal nerve, itself a branch of the fourth sacral nerve.

Anatomically, where would you find the anorectal junction?

This is the point where the rectum angles forward as it passes through the sling of puborectalis.

What is the dentate line?

Approximately 2 cm from the anal verge, there is a transition from the smooth non-keratinized squamous epithelium (with no hair follicles or sebaceous glands) below to the columnar intestinal epithelium above. It is notable that below the dentate line, the mucosa of the anus is very sensitive and is supplied by the inferior rectal branches of the pudendal nerve. This is important to remember when banding or performing injection sclerotherapy for haemorrhoidal disease.

What are haemorrhoids (internal piles) and in which positions are they commonly found?

Haemorrhoids are formed by enlargement of the anal cushions. The anal cushions are small submucous masses comprising fibroelastic connective tissue, smooth muscle, dilated venous spaces and arteriovenous anastamoses. They are present at 3, 7 and 11 o'clock positions in the upper anal canal.

What is the lymphatic drainage of the anal canal?

Upper third	drains to the rectal lymphatics,
Lower two-thirds	drains into the superficial inguinal nodes.

What is the neurological supply to the internal and external anal sphincter?

External sphincter	Inferior rectal branches of the pudendal nerve (sensory); Onuf's nucleus, anterior horn of S2 (motor).
Internal sphincter	Sympathetic fibres from the pelvic plexus cause contraction; parasympathetic cause relaxation.

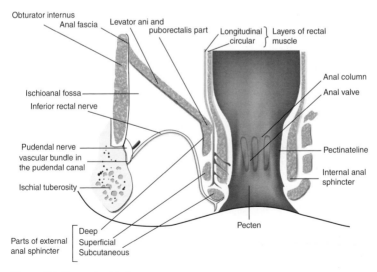

Figure 7.1 The anal sphincter.

The liver

Label Figure 7.2, using the following list

1. Lesser omentum,
2. Falciform ligament,
3. Ligamentum teres,
4. Porta hepatis,
5. Upper layer of coronary ligament,
6. Lower layer of coronary ligament,
7. Right triangular ligament,
8. Left triangular ligament,
9. Left lobe,
10. Caudate lobe,
11. Quadrate lobe,
12. IVC,
13. Gallbladder.

Answers: A-8; B-2, C-10, D-12, E-5, G-7, H-13, I-6, J-4, K-11, L-3, M-1, N-9.

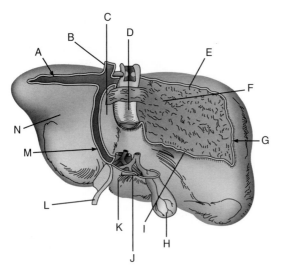

Figure 7.2
Peritoneal reflections on the posterior (visceral surface) of the liver.

What are the surface markings of the liver?

Superior margin –– Xiphisternum to the fifth intercostal space (ICS), approximately 7–8 cm from the midline on the left and the fifth rib on the right.

Right –– The seventh to eleventh ribs in a mid-axillary line.

Inferior margin –– Approximately along the right costal margin passing a hand's breadth below the xiphisternum to meet the leftmost point of the superior margin at the left fifth ICS.

How do the functional and anatomical divisions of the liver differ?

Anatomically, the liver is divided into the right and left lobes by the falciform ligament anteriorly and the fissures of the ligamentum teres and the ligamentum venosum posteriorly. Functionally, the liver is divided in accordance to its blood supply along the plane in which the middle hepatic vein lies. This corresponds to an oblique line running through the centre of the gallbladder bed and the groove of the IVC.

Is there communication between the vascular supplies to the left and right lobes of the liver?

No. These are end arteries. However, in the presence of disease, collaterals may develop in the bare area with the phrenic vessels.

Briefly describe the extra-hepatic biliary tree

The right and left hepatic ducts leave the liver and join to form the common hepatic duct at the porta hepatis. The common hepatic duct passes between the two layers of peritoneum in the free edge of the lesser omentum and is joined by the cystic duct from the gallbladder to form the common bile duct (CBD). The CBD enters the second part of the duodenum with the pancreatic duct at the ampulla of Vater (hepatopancreatic ampulla).

What is the capacity of the gallbladder?

Approximately 30–50 ml.

What is Hartmann's pouch?

This is a small diverticulum in the wall of the neck of the gallbladder where it joins the cystic duct. This may be the site of an impacted gallstone.

What are the borders of Calot's triangle? What is its significance?

This is the triangle formed by the liver, the common hepatic duct and the cystic duct. The cystic artery runs across it. The cystic node also lies within it at the junction of the cystic and common hepatic ducts.

What is the maximum normal diameter of the common bile duct?

6 mm. It may be larger postcholecystectomy.

What are the three parts of the common bile duct?

First part In the free edge of the lesser omentum at the entry to the lesser sac,

Second part Posterior to the first part of the duodenum,

Third part Grooves the posterior aspect of the head of the pancreas and the second part of the duodenum.

What is Pringle's manoeuvre?

This is when the free edge of the lesser omentum (i.e., the CBD, common hepatic artery and portal vein) is compressed between the thumb and forefinger (or by clamp) to temporarily control haemorrhage from the liver.

What is the blood supply to the pancreas?

Head Superior and inferior pancreaticoduodenal arteries,

Neck, body and tail Splenic artery.

Briefly describe the two peritoneal attachments of the spleen

Gastrosplenic ligament: Formed from the peritoneum passing from the hilum of the spleen to the greater curvature of the stomach.

Splenorenal ligament: Formed from the leaves of peritoneum reflecting backwards to the front of the left kidney. The splenic artery passes between the two leaves of the splenorenal ligament.

Chapter

8

Applied surgical physiology

Swallowing

What volume of saliva is normally produced per day?

0.5–1.0 litres.

Where is saliva produced?

1. Submandibular glands (70% saliva produced here): opens into oral cavity via Wharton's duct at a small papilla lateral to the frenulum linguae; supplied by the facial nerve.

2. Parotid gland: opens into oral cavity adjacent to the second molar tooth via Stensen's duct; supplied by the glossopharyngeal nerve.

3. Saliva is also produced by the sublingual and minor salivary glands within the oral mucosa.

By which neurological mechanisms is the secretion of saliva controlled?

The parasympathetic nervous system stimulates the secretion of profuse watery saliva. The sympathetic system stimulates thick, mucinous saliva secretion.

What are the three phases of swallowing?

Oral, pharyngeal and oesophageal phases.

Describe the mechanisms involved in the oral phase of swallowing

This is initiated voluntarily after chewing food. After chewing, the rolling action of the tongue against the hard palate pushes the food bolus upwards and backwards. On sensation of the food bolus at the posterior pharynx, the involuntary pharyngeal phase is initiated.

Describe the mechanisms involved in the pharyngeal phase

The sensation of food bolus in the posterior pharynx stimulates sensory afferents in the glossopharyngeal and vagus nerves, which stimulate the medullary *swallowing centre*. Efferent impulses in the same nerves reflexively trigger swallowing and respiration is simultaneously inhibited.

- Initially, the superior constrictor contracts, elevating the soft palate and preventing food from entering the nasopharynx.
- Contraction of palatopharyngeus narrows the aperture of the pharynx and prevents further food from entering.
- The true vocal folds now come together and the larynx is elevated against the epiglottis. This prevents aspiration and opens the oesophagus.
- The upper oesophageal sphincter then relaxes and the superior constrictor contracts, forcing the bolus into the oesophagus.

Describe the mechanisms involved in the oesophageal phase

Entry of the food bolus into the oesophagus initiates the primary peristaltic wave. The lower oesophageal sphincter simultaneously relaxes. If remaining food bolus is sensed within the oesophagus, the secondary peristaltic wave is initiated, beginning at the site of distension.

What is the normal resting pressure of the lower oesophageal sphincter (LOS)?

30 mmHg.

Which structures make up the LOS?

There is no distinct anatomical sphincter in the lower oesophagus. The LOS is made up of a combination of anatomical and physiological elements that together maintain a zone of high pressure in the lower oesophagus and prevent reflux. These include:

- The intrinsic muscles of the distal oesophagus: contract to prevent reflux when swallowing is not taking place.
- The right crus of the diaphragm: acts like a sling around the lower oesophagus.
- The mucosal folds within the oesophagus: provide a valve-like function.
- The acute angle of entry of the oesophagus into the stomach: provides a valve-like function.
- The intra-abdominal pressure: compresses the intra-abdominal portion of the oesophagus.

Defecation

What are the mechanisms involved in maintaining normal continence?

- Contraction of puborectalis: maintains the angle between the rectum and the anal canal.
- Contraction of the external anal sphincter (voluntary, cortical control).

- Involuntary tonic contractions of the internal anal sphincter.
- 'Flutter valve' mechanism: abdominal pressure results in flattening of the mid to lower anterior rectal wall, occluding it and preventing distal transit of rectal contents.
- Anal mucosal cushions: provide a further mechanism to provide a tight seal to prevent faecal leakage.

Briefly explain the intrinsic mechanisms involved in defecation

Stretch receptors in the rectal wall are stimulated on entry of faeces into the rectum. Afferent signals from the myenteric plexus initiate peristalsis in the descending colon, sigmoid and rectum, and force faeces towards the anus. At the same time, the puborectalis relaxes, reducing the angle between the rectum and the anus. Distension of the rectum leads to reflex relaxation of the internal anal sphincter (the *recto-anal inhibitory reflex*). At this point, if there is a simultaneous voluntary release of cortical inhibition on the external sphincter this also relaxes, leading to defecation. If the circumstances for defecation are unfavourable, the external anal sphincter contracts and the rectum and sigmoid relax until the next bolus of faecal material is propelled into the rectum.

What role do spinal cord reflexes play in defecation?

The *intrinsic (myenteric) reflex* alone is relatively weak and, therefore, the parasympathetic spinal cord reflex plays a key role in defecation. Distension of the rectum also sends afferent signals to the sacral cord. From here impulses travel via preganglionic parasympathetic fibres in the pelvic nerves to the descending colon, sigmoid and rectum, where they synapse with postganglionic fibres and stimulate contraction, intensifying peristalsis. Afferent signals entering the spinal cord also initiate the Valsalva manoeuvre and contraction of the abdominal muscles adding force to defecation by increasing intra-abdominal pressure.

Which spinal levels are involved in the defecation reflex?

Both sensory and motor fibres originate from S2 to S4.

Micturition

What is the capacity of the bladder?

Approximately 500 ml.

At what volume is the first urge to micturate felt?

At about 150 ml. At 400 ml, a marked sense of fullness is felt.

Autonomic supply to the bladder is from which spinal levels?

Sympathetic -- L1–L3. These fibres travel with the hypogastric nerves. Contraction of the sphincter is α_1 mediated, relaxation of the detrusor is β_2 mediated.

Parasympathetic -- S2–S4. The parasympathetic system leads to contraction of the detrusor and relaxation of the sphincter.

What are the key aspects of the sphincter mechanism in the male and female?

In both the male and female, a combination between the bladder neck and distal urethral sphincter mechanisms maintain urinary continence.

Male -- The bladder neck mechanism not only provides urinary continence but also prevents retrograde ejaculation. The distal sphincter mechanism lies at the base of the prostate gland within the urethra. It is capable of maintaining continence even if there is damage to the bladder neck mechanism.

Female -- The bladder neck mechanism is poorly defined. The distal sphincter mechanism maintains urinary continence and extends along two-thirds of the urethra.

What are the two phases of bladder function?

1. Storage phase,
2. Voiding phase.

What is meant by 'receptive relaxation', and when does this occur?

During the storage phase, the bladder undergoes receptive relaxation. Filling stimulates suburothelial stretch receptors, which initially induce low-frequency firing of sensory afferents in the underfilled bladder. Such low-frequency afferent signals cause relaxation of the bladder by inhibiting the parasympathetic preganglionic neurons and exciting the lumbar sympathetic preganglionic neurons. As a result, the bladder relaxes, resulting in little increase in the pressure within it (Laplace's law applies: i.e., by increasing the radius for an increased wall tension, the pressure within the vessel may be kept constant).

Briefly explain the processes involved in the storage phase of micturition

Stretch receptors in the suburothelial layer are stimulated by bladder filling and send impulses via the pelvic nerves to sacral segments of the spinal cord, initially resulting in receptive relaxation. As the bladder becomes full, afferent firing increases and filling is consciously perceived by the cortical centres. Central (voluntary) pathways act to prevent unintentional voiding by inhibiting the *pontine micturition centre*. Afferent input also stimulates a spinal reflex, causing contraction of the skeletal muscle sphincter through excitation of Onuf's nucleus, and contraction of the bladder neck and urethra through excitation of the sympathetic preganglionic neurons.

Briefly explain the processes involved in the voiding phase of micturition

Increased bladder filling increases the firing of sensory afferents and activates the *pontine micturition centre*. When the cortical inhibition is removed by the conscious decision to pass urine, maximal firing of the pontine micturition centre occurs, causing excitation of the sacral preganglionic parasympathetic neurons resulting in contraction of the detrusor muscle and a sudden increase in intravesical pressure. Impulses to *Onuf's nucleus* also cause relaxation of the distal urethral sphincter and release of urine via the urethra. Furthermore, the flow of urine through the urethra also stimulates a urethral stretch reflex, which itself stimulates contraction of the detrusor until the bladder is empty. Conscious contraction of the abdominal muscles may also aid expulsion of urine by increasing intra-abdominal pressure.

The abdominal wall

Surgical approaches to the abdomen

On Figure 9.1, label each incision and give an example of its potential indication

A. Rooftop,

B. Thoraco-abdominal,

C. Kocher's,

D. Right paramedian,

E. Midline,

F. Gridiron,

G. Lanz,

H. Pfannenstiel,

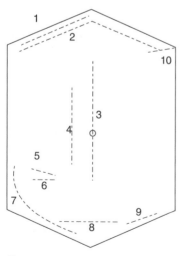

Figure 9.1 Abdominal incisions.

I. Left groin,

J. Rutherford Morrison,

Answers: 1-C, 2-A, 3-E, 4-D, 5-F, 6-G, 7-J, 8-H, 9-I, 10-B.

Rooftop	Total gastrectomy, liver transplantation
Thoraco-abdominal	Oesophagectomy
Kocher's	Open cholecystectomy, splenic surgery if on left.
Right paramedian	Renal surgery
Midline	Large and small bowel resections. Look for scars consistent with closure of stoma sites.
Pfannenstiel	Caesarean section, bladder, prostate, pelvic resections.
Left groin	Open inguinal hernia repair
Gridiron and Lanz	Open appendectomy
Rutherford Morrison	Renal transplantation

Describe how you would perform a midline laparotomy incision to gain access to the peritoneal cavity

The patient should be placed in either the supine or Lloyd Davis position, depending on the primary aim of the procedure. The position of the incision is dependent on the structures needing to be accessed. In the upper abdomen, the incision is made in the midline extending from just below the xiphoid process to the umbilicus. In the lower abdomen, the incision may begin in the supraumbilical region, passing around the umbilicus and along the midline to the suprapubic region. The incision first passes through the skin and subcutaneous fat followed by the linea alba. Finally, the peritoneum is carefully divided in the region of the umbilicus to enter the peritoneal cavity. The bladder must be carefully avoided at the inferiormost aspect of the incision (a urinary catheter should be placed prior to the start of the procedure).

What are the advantages of the midline incision?

1. It is almost bloodless,
2. No muscle fibres are divided,
3. There is little risk of neurological injury,
4. It provides good access to both upper and lower abdominal organs,
5. It is usually quick to perform and to close.

What is Jenkin's rule in closure of a midline incision?

Suture length $= 4 \times$ length of the incision.

1 cm bites of the sheath should be taken 1 cm apart.

Stomas

List the differences in external appearance of an ileostomy and colostomy

Ileostomy –– Spouted, loose 'mint sauce' contents in the stoma bag, often on the right side of the abdomen (although not always), may be associated with surrounding skin irritation (as ileostomy effluent contains proteolytic enzymes and bile salts that corrode the surrounding skin).

Colostomy –– Flush with the skin, formed faeculant stool within the stoma bag, often on the left side of the abdomen.

What features would you look for when examining a stoma?

- Contents: urine, formed or liquid stool.
- Loop or end? Digitate the stoma to examine the opening or openings. Loop stomas will have two lumina, one proximal and one distal limb.
- Is there obvious prolapse or retraction of the bowel?
- Characteristics of the mucosa: the mucosa should be warm, pink and well perfused.
- Surrounding skin: is the surrounding skin healthy or is there irritation?
- Examine for a parastomal hernia or prolapse.
- Surrounding scars: open or laparoscopic surgery, is there evidence of previous healed stoma sites, examine the perineum: Is there a perineal wound that would indicate an abdomino-perineal resection?

What are the complications of stoma formation?

Immediate or early –– Ischaemia, bleeding, infection, skin excoriation, dehydration, electrolyte disturbance and nutritional deficiency following high output.

Late –– Prolapse, fistulation, retraction, parastomal hernia, skin excoriation, stenosis, recurrence of disease and electrolyte or nutritional deficiencies.

List the key indications for stoma formation

Diversion	To protect a distal anastomosis (e.g., loop ileostomy following large bowel resection) or urinary diversion following cystectomy.

Exteriorization	In the presence of contamination (where primary anastomosis has a high risk of breakdown), or for permanent terminalization of the colon or ileum (e.g., following AP resection).
Decompression	In the setting of intestinal obstruction to prior to definitive treatment of the cause of obstruction.

Temporary or permanent exteriorization following resection is the main absolute indication for stoma formation. The others listed are relative and may depend on the surgeon's preference and experience.

Inguinal herniae

Define the borders of the inguinal canal

Floor	Inguinal ligament,
Roof	Lower border of internal oblique and transversus abdominis muscles,
Anteriorly	External oblique aponeurosis,
Posterior wall	Transversalis fascia throughout and conjoint tendon medially.

What is the surface marking of the deep ring?

The deep ring is approximately 1 cm above the midpoint of the inguinal ligament, which is halfway along a line joining the pubic tubercle to the anterior superior iliac spine (ASIS).

What is the difference between the midpoint of the inguinal ligament and the mid inguinal point?

The midpoint of the inguinal ligament is midway along a line joining the ASIS and the pubic tubercule. This is the landmark for the deep ring. The mid inguinal point is midway along a line joining the ASIS and the pubic symphysis. This is the surface landmark of the femoral pulse.

Which structures pass through the deep inguinal ring?

1. Spermatic cord (vas deferens, testicular artery and veins and cremasteric artery) or round ligament of the uterus in the female,
2. Genital branch of the genitofemoral nerve,
3. Autonomic nerves and lymphatics.

How does the ilioinguinal nerve enter and leave the inguinal canal and which structures does it innervate?

The ilioinguinal nerve pierces the internal oblique to enter the inguinal canal; it leaves the canal via the superficial ring. Its innervation is to the skin overlying the inguinal region, upper thigh, root of the penis and anterior scrotum. In the female, it supplies sensation to the labium majus.

What are the boundaries of Hasselbach's triangle?

Medial	Lateral border of the rectus muscle,
Laterally	Inferior epigastric artery,
Floor	Conjoint tendon and fascia transversalis,
Inferiorly	Inguinal ligament.

What is the significance of this region?

It is the site of a direct inguinal hernia.

What are the key points to demonstrate in examining an inguinal hernia?

1. Inspect the region and identify the lump. Describe its position and general appearance. Remark on any overlying skin changes.
2. Define the anatomy and demonstrate that the lump arises from above the inguinal ligament (i.e., it is not a femoral hernia).
3. Demonstrate a palpable cough impulse (start with the patient standing up and the hernia reduced, then move on to examine it with the patient lying down).
4. Ask the patient to reduce the hernia if possible. If this is possible, with the hernia reduced occlude the deep ring and ask the patient to cough again. An indirect hernia will be controlled by pressure over the deep ring, a direct hernia will not (it is, however, worth mentioning that this test is notoriously unreliable and definitive classification can only be noted at the time of surgery).

Describe the Lichtenstein technique of inguinal hernia repair

With the patient in the supine position, an oblique groin incision is made and extended through skin and subcutaneous fat and fascia until the external oblique aponeurosis is identified. The external oblique is entered and the spermatic cord is identified and dissected free from the posterior wall of the inguinal canal. A tape may be placed around the cord at this stage. The hernial sac is then identified as either indirect or direct. In the case of an indirect sac, this is dissected free from the cord and dissected back to the deep ring. The sac is then opened and the contents inspected before being reduced. The sac may then be ligated and the distal sac excised if small (a large inguino-scrotal sac may be left open to prevent hydrocele formation). In the case of a direct hernia, the sac is identified and either reduced or plicated. A polypropylene mesh is cut to fit the inguinal canal and the apex is either sutured or tacked to the pubic tubercle. The lower border of the mesh is then either sutured (continuous prolene) or tacked to the edge of the inguinal ligament and the medial border is secured to the conjoint tendon. The tails of the mesh are then secured around the spermatic cord to create the new superficial ring. Haemostasis is then ensured and the external oblique closed with continuous absorbable sutures. Subcutaneous tissues are approximated and skin closed with a subcuticular suture.

What are the indications for laparoscopic inguinal hernia repair?

Historically, laparoscopic inguinal hernia repair was only recommended in bilateral or recurrent herniae. However, current NICE guidelines state that laparoscopic inguinal hernia repair should be considered as a potential treatment option for all inguinal herniae and patients should be 'fully informed of all the risks and benefits of open and laparoscopic surgery by either the TAPP or TEP, to enable them to choose between the procedures' (NICE guidance TA83, September 2004). Previous abdominal surgery, cardiopulmonary disease limiting pneumoperitoneum, incarcerated or irreducible herniae are relative contraindications to laparoscopic repair.

Which options are available in laparoscopic inguinal hernia repair?

TAPP (transabdominal preperitoneal) repair –– The peritoneal cavity is entered by insertion of a 10 or 12 mm umbilical port and two further ports (site dependent on the side of the hernia). A general laparoscopy is initially performed and both groins are examined. The anatomy and defect is then identified and the contents of the hernia gently reduced with the atraumatic grasper. A preperitoneal flap is created by incising the peritoneum approx 4 cm lateral to the deep ring to the pubis medially. The contents are dissected free from the sac and the sac may be ligated at this stage. Laparoscopic mesh is then rolled and inserted via the umbilical port. The mesh may then be secured by tacking to the pubic bone and Cooper's ligament medially, and to at least 2–3 cm beyond the deep ring laterally (note: some laparoscopic specific meshes do not require tacking). After fixing the mesh, the peritoneal flap is closed over the mesh with a layer of continuous sutures.

TEP (total extraperitoneal) repair –– The TEP repair involves creation of the preperitoneal space. An infraumbilical incision is made and dissection extended to the anterior rectus sheath. The anterior rectus sheath is entered and the recti retracted to expose the posterior rectus sheath. The balloon dissector (spacemaker) is then placed into the plane just anterior to the posterior rectus sheath and the laparoscope inserted. At the same time, the balloon dissector is manually insufflated, and the preperitoneal space created. The balloon dissector is then withdrawn and the gas connected to the port to insufflate the preperitoneal space. Further laparoscopic ports may now be inserted in the midline – 10 mm halfway between the umbilicus and pubis, and 5 mm approximately 5 cm above the pubis. The inferior epigastric vessels should be identified and traced to the deep ring. The hernial sac is then visualized and the dissection made around the sac. The cord structures are then dissected free from the sac. The rolled laparoscopic mesh is then inserted via the umbilical port (as in the TAPP repair), and fixed superiorly approximately 3 cm above the internal ring. Once the mesh is in place, the area is examined prior to removal of the balloon dissector and ports. The anterior rectus sheath is closed with absorbable sutures. It is worth noting that if the peritoneum is breached during the TEP repair the inadvertent creation of pneumoperitoneum impairs visualization of structures and may require conversion to a TAPP approach.

What are the complications commonly associated with laparoscopic hernia repair?

Immediate –– Urinary retention, injury to vas, nerve injury, inadvertent bowel injury, vascular injury to iliac, inferior epigastric or spermatic vessels resulting in either severe acute haemorrhage or groin or scrotal haematoma formation.

Early –– Seroma, infection, ischaemic orchitis, testicular atrophy, pain, anastomotic leak in the case of bowel resection.

Late –– Adhesions and intestinal obstruction, hernia recurrence, migration of mesh.

What is the 'triangle of doom'?

The 'triangle of doom' is the area bordered laterally by the spermatic vessels, medially by the vas deferens and its apex at the deep inguinal ring. This external iliac artery and vein run through here and tacking of the mesh in this area should therefore be avoided.

What is the 'triangle of pain'?

The 'triangle of pain' is the area bounded medially by the spermatic vessels, and superolaterally by the iliopubic tract. In this area, tacking of the mesh should be avoided due to the risk of injury to the lateral femoral cutaneous nerve or the femoral branch of the genitofemoral nerve.

Which nerves are at particular risk during laparoscopic inguinal hernia repair?

Damage to the lateral cutaneous nerve of the thigh and the femoral branch of the genitofemoral nerve may occur due to lateral placement of tacks when securing the mesh. Injury to the lateral femoral cutaneous nerve may result in pain, paraesthesia or hyperaesthesia of the upper thigh and hip. Genitofemoral nerve injury results in similar symptoms in the skin over the scrotum. This is usually self-limiting.

Femoral herniae

What are the borders of the femoral canal?

Anteriorly	Inguinal ligament,
Posteriorly	Pectineal ligament,
Medially	Lacunar ligament,
Laterally	Femoral vein.

What are the key clinical features of a femoral hernia?

1. On examination, the lump is palpable below the inguinal ligament.
2. The lump is medial to the femoral pulse.
3. The lump is inferior and lateral to the pubic tubercle.
4. It is usually irreducible without a palpable cough impulse. Most femoral herniae are repaired on an urgent or emergent basis as the risk of strangulation is high.
5. Femoral herniae are more common in women than in men (2:1) although inguinal herniae are more common than femoral herniae in both men and women.

Which surgical approaches to femoral herniae repair are available? Briefly describe each

Several approaches have been described. These include the Lockwood (low), Lotheissen (transinguinal) and McEvedy (high) approach.

Lockwood –– This is the most common approach. The incision is placed directly over the hernia below the inguinal ligament. The sac is then identified, dissected free, opened and the contents inspected and reduced. The sac is then ligated and the defect closed. Repair may be performed by means of a mesh plug, which is inserted into the femoral canal and secured to the inguinal ligament anteriorly, the pectineal ligament posteriorly and the lacunar ligament medially. Alternatively, the inguinal ligament and pectineal ligament may be approximated and sutured with a non-absorbable suture.

Lotheissen (preperitoneal) –– This may be used when the aetiology of the hernia is uncertain, as inguinal herniae may also be repaired without an additional incision. The incision is made 2.5 cm above the medial half of the inguinal ligament and extended through the external oblique into the inguinal canal. The external ring is then identified and the spermatic cord (or round ligament) isolated and freed from the posterior wall of the canal (as in an inguinal hernia repair). An incision is made in the posterior wall of the inguinal canal to expose the femoral canal from above. The sac is then visualized and freed from surrounding tissue. Reduction of the sac may require division of the lacunar ligament. The sac is opened, the contents inspected and reduced and the sac transfixed and ligated, as previously described. Repair may then be carried out by means of a mesh plug or direct approximation of the inguinal and pectineal ligaments.

McEvedy –– This is used in emergency setting in the case of a strangulated hernia likely to require bowel resection. A transverse incision is made approximately 5 cm above the inguinal ligament. After dissecting through the subcutaneous tissues, a vertical incision is made in the rectus sheath just lateral to the lateral border of the rectus muscle to expose the peritoneum. Blunt dissection is performed to the femoral ring to expose the neck of the hernial sac. After identifying the sac, it is then dissected free and reduced. If the sac is not reducible, the lacunar ligament may need to be divided. The sac is then opened and the contents inspected. Provided that the contents are viable, they are reduced and the sac transfixed and ligated. Repair may then be performed by means of a mesh plug or direct approximation of the inguinal and pectineal ligaments, as previously described.

Umbilical and paraumbilical herniae

What is the difference between a true umbilical hernia and a paraumbilical hernia?

True umbilical herniae –– These are through the umbilical scar and may be present from childhood. Spontaneous occurrence is uncommon in adults and may be secondary to pregnancy, ascites, ovarian or uterine pathology.

Paraumbilical herniae –– These are more common in males, those of Afro-Caribbean origin and with obesity. The hernia occurs due to a defect in the linea alba, adjacent to the umbilical scar. These herniae usually contain preperitoneal fat; however, the defect is often small and there is a high risk of strangulation if bowel is contained within the hernial sac).

What are the surgical options in open repair of paraumbilical herniae?

The emphasis should be placed on a 'tension-free' repair to reduce the risk of recurrence. Either the Mayo technique (direct closure overlapping the two edges of the rectus) may be used or a mesh placed.

Mayo technique –– Either an infraumbilical or a supraumbilical incision is made, and the dissection continued down to the rectus sheath, which is exposed around the region of the defect. The sac is freed and the umbilicus disconnected if necessary. The sac should be opened, the contents inspected and reduced if healthy. The sac is then ligated and excised completely. The lower edge of one side of the rectus sheath is then overlapped with the upper edge of the other side by means of mattress sutures. A second layer of interrupted sutures is then used to secure the anterior edge in place. The umbilicus is repositioned if necessary prior to closure.

Mesh repair –– The approach to the hernial sac is as described. Once the contents have been reduced and the sac ligated, a suitable mesh (e.g., polypropylene) is cut to the appropriate size and positioned over the defect. A clear margin of at least 2–3 cm around the defect should be ensured to reduce the risk of recurrence. The mesh is then fixed in position with interrupted non-absorbable sutures and closure performed, as previously described.

The abdominal aorta and abdominal aortic aneurysms

What is the commonest site of aneurysm formation?

Prior to the discovery of penicillin, the most common type of aortic aneurysm was of the aortic arch secondary to syphilis. However, in modern practice the infrarenal abdominal aorta (see Figure 10.1) is the most commonly affected. The most common peripheral aneurysmal artery is the popliteal artery.

How may aneurysmal dilatation of the aorta be classified?

By convention, aortic aneurysms are divided into:

1. Ascending and descending thoracic aortic aneurysms (TAA),
2. Thoraco-abdominal aortic aneurysms,
3. Suprarenal aortic aneurysms (involving the renal arteries, coeliac axis and the superior mesenteric artery – the visceral segment),
4. Juxtarenal aortic aneurysms (the aneurysm starts below the renal arteries, but necessitates clamping above them),
5. Infrarenal aortic aneurysms.

What is the prevalence of AAA?

Approximately 7–8% of men over the age of 65 years have an AAA. In the USA, 32 000 AAA repairs are performed yearly, with 105 000 patients receiving a diagnosis of AAA. This compares with an incidence of 10 per 100 000 patients yearly for TAA. About 75% of all aneurysm repairs are of the abdominal aorta with the vast majority being elective procedures (62.3% vs. 12.7%).

Aneurysmal disease is multifocal: 12% of patients with AAA having a TAA, and 50% of those with a TAA have a further aneurysm.

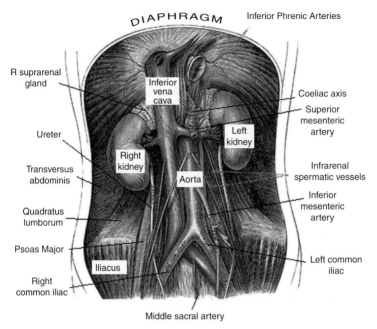

Figure 10.1 The abdominal aorta. Reproduced from Henry Gray. (1918) *Anatomy of the Human Body.*

What is the aetiology of abdominal aortic aneurysms (AAA)?

Degeneration –– Most AAAs are the result of an incompletely understood complex degenerative process. This has previously been called atherosclerosis, but is distinct from other atherosclerotic occlusive disease, as there is no typically significant occlusion disease. Whilst atherosclerosis is a feature of aneurysmal disease it is not clear whether this is a causative or reactionary factor. Extensive research is ongoing to find the true cause.

Inflammation –– This is associated with the condition retroperitoneal fibrosis, which also affects the ureters and leads to encasement in a thick inflammatory tissue mass. It is currently thought that these two conditions are part of the same spectrum of disease, and that all AAAs have an element of inflammation in their formation. Rheumatological vasculitides can also be associated with aneurysms.

Post-dissection –– Following dissection, the outer wall of the false lumen can degenerate and lead to the formation of a true aneurysm.

Trauma –– Aneurysms due to trauma are, by definition, false aneurysms.

Infection –– Classically, these are called 'mycotic' aneurysms, though many are not secondary to fungal infections. Infections can cause primary aneurysms and also infect pre-existing aneurysms. Infection of a prosthetic graft can lead to breakdown of the anastomosis between tissue and graft, leading to rupture, or to graft thrombosis.

What are the risk factors for developing AAA?

Numerous risk factors have been found for AAA development including advanced age, cigarette smoking, family history, hypertension, male sex, obesity, hypercholesterolaemia, and the presence of atherosclerotic occlusive disease, such as coronary artery occlusive disease. The most significant of these are smoking and male sex – a relative risk of $5.6\times$ and $4.5\times$, respectively.

What proportion of AAAs are asymptomatic?

Approximately 75%.

Briefly describe the physiological mechanism behind expansion of AAA

This expansion is due to Laplace's law – the larger the vessel radius, the larger the wall tension (T) required to withstand a given internal fluid pressure. This is governed by the pressure difference across the wall (P – blood pressure), the vessel radius (R), and vessel wall thickness (M). This gives the equation

$$T = (P \times R)/M.$$

From this, it is easy to see that as the vessel becomes more aneurysmal and the wall gets stretched (and therefore thinner), the wall tension increases dramatically. Therefore, larger aneurysms expand more quickly.

How are AAAs diagnosed?

Usually, AAAs are diagnosed on clinical examination, though this is notoriously inaccurate, with approximately 50% of aneurysms of operable size not clinically palpable. Duplex ultrasound (B-mode ultrasound combined with colour Doppler flow measurements) and computed tomography (CT) with contrast are the gold standard tests. The combination of two modalities allows ultrasound to be used for detection and monitoring, with CT reserved for measurements and planning purposes, therefore reducing the patient's radiation load.

Most AAAs are found incidentally, when the patient has imaging for other causes. Currently a national screening programme is being implemented and rolled out across the UK. This aims to use ultrasound scanning to screen all men in the year that they turn 65.

What are the symptoms associated with AAA?

Though often asymptomatic until rupture, AAAs may cause the following symptoms:

1. Chronic back pain,
2. Compressive symptoms on surrounding structures (if large),
3. Emboli – due to the expansion in the lumen of the vessel, slower flow areas develop at the vessel walls. This leads to thrombus formation, which can cause distal embolization and acutely ischaemic limbs, and, rarely, complete aortic occlusion. Thus, if an ischaemic leg is found, an AAA must be excluded.

If an AAA becomes painful at rest or tender on palpation this is a sign of impending rupture and necessitates expedited repair.

What features may be associated with rupture of an AAA?

The classic triad:

1. Severe abdominal or back pain,
2. Hypotension,
3. Palpable pulsatile mass.

In addition:

4. Groin or loin pain, sometimes mimicking testicular torsion or renal colic,
5. Generalized abdominal peritonitis: due to rupture into the peritoneal cavity.

How does the risk of rupture of AAA vary with aneurysm size?

Size of AAA (cm)	Risk of rupture per year (%)
<3.0	0
3–3.9	0.4
4–4.9	1.1
5–5.9	3.3
6–6.9	9.4
7–7.9	24

What are the features of AAA rupture?

If the arterial wall is breached, the rupture is temporarily controlled by two factors – the weak posterior parietal peritoneum and the hypotension caused by bleeding into the retroperitoneum. It is at this stage that successful repair can be undertaken. Successful repair depends on specialized high volume surgeons and centres equipped for rAAA surgery. There is currently a move to reorganize vascular services into centralized tertiary centres.

What is the prognosis of rAAA?

Ruptured AAA has a high mortality rate: 50% reach hospital, 50% of those reach theatre and 50% of those survive, giving a survival rate of approximately 12.5%. In comparison, elective mortality rates for vascular centres are 1–5%.

Note: even with successful elective repair, the five-year survival is approximately 65%, compared with 85% in matched controls.

What surgical strategies are available in the management of AAA?

1. Endovascular repair,
2. Open repair.

Briefly describe the open surgical management of AAA

This may be via a traditional open or laparoscopic approach, which may be transperitoneal or retroperitoneal (far less common).

Transperitoneal approach to infrarenal AAA –– A midline laparotomy incision is made, and the small bowel is mobilized, retracted and protected. The aneurysm sac is identified. The posterior peritoneum overlying the aorta is incised from bifurcation to the ligament of Treitz, with mobilization of the left renal vein (which will cross in front of the aorta in most cases, but can cross behind). Systemic heparin is given and the infrarenal aorta is cross-clamped. Clamps are then applied to the common iliac arteries, with careful preservation of the ureters. The aneurysm is then opened, the underlying thrombus removed and interior of the sac examined. The lumbar arteries branching off the aorta are then ligated with non-absorbable sutures, and if the inferior mesenteric artery is not occluded, it too can be ligated (blood supply to the bowel is protected by the collateral supply). A Dacron graft is then anastamosed to the infrarenal aorta and then subsequently to the distal aorta or iliac arteries, using non-absorbable sutures. This is called 'endoaneurysmorrhaphy'. The aneurysmal sac and posterior peritoneum are then closed to provide good tissue barriers between the duodenum and the graft, to prevent an aortoduodenal fistula.

Briefly describe the endovascular technique in management of an infrarenal AAA

The basic principle of endovascular aneurysm repair (EVAR) is the same as any endovascular technique – Seldinger technique access under fluoroscopic guidance with contrast for adequate deployment of the graft. The EVAR grafts are Dacron reinforced with a self-expanding stent. Endovascular treatment necessitates CT with contrast for stent planning, leading to 'bespoke' designs, with multiple modules. Access to the aorta is normally gained via the femoral arteries, with complicated stents requiring brachial or carotid artery access. This access is via either percutaneous needle puncture or bilateral femoral artery cutdowns. Once access to the femoral artery is gained, a guidewire is fed under fluoroscopic guidance to the aorta. An access sheath (allowing easy exchange of wires, catheters and the stent) is then placed and exact positioning of stent graft is accomplished using contrast injections. The stent graft is then deployed in modular fashion. Pre- and postdeployment angiographic contrast runs are completed to ensure positioning and prevention of leak around the stent sealing points.

What is the difference between open repair of AAA (oAAA) and EVAR?

Open repair offers a procedure that once completed needs little follow-up. It has extensive evidence backing the management and long-term outcomes. No further imaging is required in most cases. However, it has a significant physiological impact with an intensive care unit stay required postoperatively. In contrast, EVAR has a much lower physiological impact, with 48-hour bed stays possible (and in some cases 24 hours) but it does necessitate lifelong follow-up and stent imaging. However, we have little long-term outcome data on EVAR, owing to extensive developments in the technique since its conception. The EVAR 1 and EVAR 2 trials have shown equivalence in long-term mortality and morbidity, with short-term benefits for EVAR, being matched by fewer long-term complications for oAAA. This allows patient selection and physician and patient choice to inform management decisions.

What are the procedure-specific complications associated with repair of AAA?

Early –– Abdominal compartment syndrome after rAAA, due to retroperitoneal haematoma and inflammation; renal failure; respiratory failure; stroke; MI and death.

Late –– Anastomotic dilatation, endoleak (leak around an EVAR graft), EVAR graft migration, and rarely graft rupture.

The oesophagus, stomach and small bowel

Gastric and duodenal ulceration

Which underlying aetiological factors have been associated with peptic ulcer disease?

Helicobacter pylori infection –– Colonizes the entire gastric epithelium and causes increased gastric acid secretion by producing ammonia, which locally suppresses somatostatin inhibition of gastrin release by antral D cells. *H. pylori* also disrupts mucosal integrity by release of proteases and phospholipases.

Non-steroidal anti-inflammatory drugs (NSAIDs) –– Inhibit cyclo-oxygenase and decrease prostoglandin production. Prostaglandins (E type) act to increase both mucosal blood flow and the production of mucus and bicarbonate, which form a protective layer and act as a buffer for gastric acid, respectively. There is a dose-dependent relationship. Selective Cox-2 inhibitors have been shown to lower the risk of gastric ulceration but do not eliminate this risk.

Smoking –– May cause duodenal ulceration by increasing gastric emptying and decreasing pancreatic bicarbonate production.

Gastrinoma (Zollinger–Ellison syndrome) –– This results in hypersecretion of gastric acid and significant disruption of mucosal integrity. Ulcers may occur in both the stomach and duodenum and are often multiple.

Drugs –– For example, 5-fluorouracil, methotrexate, cyclophosphamide, spironolactone and bisphosphonates.

Stress ulceration –– In severe systemic disease, e.g., burns, sepsis, multi-organ failure and cerebral trauma.

How does the mechanism of *H. pylori* infection associated with duodenal ulceration differ from that in gastric ulceration?

H. pylori does not directly colonize the duodenum: its effect in increasing the risk of duodenal ulceration is therefore indirect. Antral colonization with

H. pylori leads to a pro-inflammatory state and the production of pro-inflammatory cytokines (e.g., IL-8 and IL-1β). This increases gastrin production from G cells and inhibits somatostatin from antral D cells. Increased gastric acid secretion has an overflow effect on the duodenal epithelium and results in gastric metaplasia. These islands of gastric metaplasia may then be colonized with *H. pylori* and cause secondary mucosal damage.

How does the pain of gastric ulceration differ from that of duodenal ulceration?

Pain	Gastric ulceration	Duodenal ulceration
Site	Epigastric	Epigastric May radiate to the back (differential: pancreatic pain)
Timing		Worse at night
Relation to food	Pain worse after food	Improves initially after food Pain usually occurs 2–3 hours after food May be associated with feeling of hunger
Relieving factors	Minimal relief from antacid therapy	Often relieved with antacids

Which clinical features may be associated with complications of peptic ulcer disease?

- Nausea, vomiting or weight loss may indicate the presence of malignancy,
- Fullness, bloating, early satiety and evidence of a succussion splash on examination may be associated with gastric outlet obstruction,
- Perforation may present with epigastric guarding, rebound or generalized peritonitis,
- Acute haemorrhage may present with melaena or haematemesis and may cause hypovolaemic shock.

Which investigative tests may be used in the diagnosis of peptic ulceration?

Blood tests -- Assessment for anaemia, iron deficiency, rarely serum *H. pylori* antibody testing.

Radiological -- Double contrast barium swallow: accuracy in diagnosis is good in both gastric and duodenal ulceration but histological diagnosis cannot be given, as no biopsy may be obtained.

Endoscopy –– Visualization of ulceration and biopsy; therapeutic intervention for bleeding ulceration.

Briefly describe the methods available for *H. pylori* testing

These include:

Urea breath testing –– The patient is asked to swallow an oral solution containing carbon labelled urea. Urease produced by *H. pylori* results in the release of radiolabelled carbon. This can then be detected as radiolabelled carbon dioxide in the exhaled air.

Serum H. pylori antibody testing –– Cannot differentiate between past exposure and active infection.

H. pylori stool antigen
Endoscopic biopsy and histological detection of the bacterium or urease testing of the biopsy sample –– In the *CLO (Campylobacter-like organism) test*, a gastric antral biopsy is taken and placed in a urea-based medium containing phenol red (or another pH indicator). *H. pylori* produces urease, which hydrolyses urea to ammonia, raising the pH of the medium, and turning the specimen from yellow to red. In the absence of *H. pylori*, the specimen remains yellow – indicating a negative result.

Note –– In duodenal ulceration, non-invasive methods of *H. pylori* testing have been validated for use in confirmation of healing. In gastric ulceration, however, healing should be confirmed endoscopically and biopsies taken to exclude malignancy.

What is the commonest site of benign gastric ulceration?

At the junction of the fundus and the antrum, along the lesser curve.

How does the macroscopic appearance of a benign ulcer differ from that of a malignant ulcer?

Benign –– Discrete, punched-out ulcer with fibrinoid exudate. Usually well circumscribed with a smooth, regular, rounded edge and a flat base.

Malignant –– Often have irregular heaped up margins. The mass usually protrudes into the lumen.

Outline the key aspects involved in the pharmacological management of peptic ulceration

- Discontinue NSAIDs and other drugs that might precipitate ulceration (where possible).
- Reduction in acid secretion:

- H_2 antagonists (e.g., cimetidine, ranitidine) block the H_2 receptors on the parietal cell and consequently reduce acid secretion in response to histamine.
- PPIs (proton pump inhibitors) (e.g., omeprazole, lanzoprazole, pantoprazole): irreversibly block the H^+K^+ ATPase pump and inhibit acid release.
- Bismuth salts and sucralfate: improve mucosal repair. Sucralfate may also partially reduce acid secretion and suppress *H. pylori* infection.
- Prostaglandin analogues (e.g., misoprostol): may increase mucosal resistance and exert a weak acid suppressive effect.
- *H. pylori* eradication therapy (7–14 days).
- In the event of acute upper GI haemorrhage, fluid resuscitation and IV PPI infusion should be commenced.

Outline an appropriate protocol for *H. pylori* eradication therapy

H. pylori eradication involves a combination of acid inhibition and antibiotic therapy. It is important to note that gastric mucosal changes are usually fully reversible with this treatment.

Antibiotic	Two of clarythromycin, metronidazole, or amoxycillin, depending on microbial resistance profiles,
Proton pump inhibitor (PPI)	As per hospital protocol.

In areas of microbial resistance or in failure of first line therapy, bismuth containing quadruple therapy may be used. In the UK, protocols usually recommend a duration of therapy of 7 days, although in the USA, it is often continued for 14 days and has been shown to increase eradication rate by 5%.

Which endoscopic therapies are available for the treatment of visible bleeding?

Injection therapy	Adrenaline 1:10 000 dilution is used. Promotes haemostasis by both a vasoconstrictive and local tamponade effect.
Thermal coagulation	By means of heater probe, electrocautery, laser or argon coagulation or a combination of techniques.
Haemoclip or mechanical devices	

Combination therapy   Adrenaline may be used with thermal coagulation may also be used in ulcers with a visible vessel, active haemorrhage, or adherent clot.

What are the principle components of the Rockall score and what does it assess?

This is a scoring system based on endoscopic and clinical parameters and is a validated tool used in the estimation of the risk of mortality and re-bleeding in upper GI bleeding. It is based on:

Age

Score 0   <60 years,

Score 1   60–79 years,

Score 2   ≥80 years.

Shock

Score 0   No features of systemic shock,

Score 1   HR > 100 but BP > 100 systolic,

Score 2   HR >100 and BP < 100 systolic.

Co-morbidities

Score 2   Cardiac failure, ischaemic heart disease or any other major co-morbidity,

Score 3   Renal failure, liver failure or disseminated malignancy.

Diagnosis

Score 0   Mallory Weiss tear or no lesion identified,

Score 1   All other diagnoses, except,

Score 2   Upper GI malignancy.

Endoscopic features of recent haemorrhage

Score 0   None or dark spot only visible,

Score 2   Active bleeding, recent clot, blood in UGI tract or visible vessel.

What are the indications for surgical intervention in the treatment of peptic ulcer disease?

1.   Haemorrhage not controlled with medical therapy and endoscopic intervention,

2.   Perforation,

3.   Gastric outlet obstruction.

Approximately 5% of bleeding ulcers require operative intervention.

Briefly outline the technique involved in oversewing a peptic ulcer

The patient is placed in a supine position. After skin preparation and draping, an upper midline incision is made from the xiphisternum to the umbilicus. The stomach and duodenum are visualized and inspected for signs of perforation or haemorrhage. In the event of perforation, an omental patch is used to form a tension-free repair and peritoneal wash-out is performed prior to drain placement and closure. In the event of haemorrhage, the ulcer is oversewn in four quadrants with ligation of the feeding vessel both proximally and distally. Wash-out is performed and drains placed prior to closure.

What are the indications for elective surgery in peptic ulcer disease?

With the advent of pharmacological acid suppressive agents, elective procedures for peptic ulcer disease are now rare. The indications for such intervention include:

1. Intractable peptic ulcer disease despite adequate medical treatment in the absence of *H. pylori* infection,
2. Failure of the ulcer to heal after 8–12 weeks of therapy or relapse after discontinuation of therapy (relative indication),
3. Strong suspicion of malignancy.

Which elective strategies are available in the treatment of peptic ulceration?

Highly selective vagotomy (HSV) or parietal cell vagotomy –– Truncal vagotomy alone not only affects the nerve supply to the parietal and chief cells but also leads to gastric atony and stasis. Highly selective vagotomy selectively spares the coeliac and hepatic branches of the vagus nerve and spares the supply to the antrum and pylorus. This removes the need for a concomitant drainage procedure.

Truncal vagotomy and pyloroplasty –– In this procedure, after performing the truncal vagotomy, a pyloroplasty is performed, commonly using the Heineke–Miculicz or Finney technique. In the Heineke–Miculicz procedure, all layers of the pylorus are opened longitudinally and then closed transversely to produce a widening of the pylorus and improve gastric drainage. An omental patch may also be used to cover the incision. In the Finney procedure, the proximal 4 cm of the duodenum is mobilized and approximated to the antrum of the stomach with a layer of interrupted seromuscular sutures. A U-shaped full-thickness incision is then made into the lumen of the stomach, extending into the duodenum and transecting the pylorus. The posterior and anterior walls are then closed, creating a side-to-side anastomosis. This may also be covered with an omental patch.

Vagotomy and antrectomy –– The antrum of the stomach, pylorus and proximal 2 cm of duodenum are resected after ligation of the local marginal vessels and the gastric branches of the gastro-epiploic artery supplying this region. The vagal trunks are identified and divided. Reconstruction usually involves one of the following:

Billroth I procedure	Gastroduodenostomy – the remaining stomach is anastamosed directly to the remaining duodenum.
Billroth II procedure	Gastrojejunostomy – the remaining stomach is anastamosed to a loop of proximal jejunum and the duodenal stump is closed, creating a blind ending loop.

Upper GI malignancies

Which aetiological factors have been associated with gastric cancer?

Low socioeconomic class, smoking, *H. pylori* infection, diet (higher rates associated with the consumption of salted or pickled vegetables and lower rates with fresh vegetables and fruit), chronic gastric ulceration, atrophic gastritis, genetic factors (2–3× increase risk if patient has a first-degree relative with positive history of gastric cancer).

What is the commonest histological type of gastric cancer?

Adenocarcinoma, which accounts for approximately 95% of gastric neoplasms. This may be divided into

Intestinal type	Intestinal metaplasia occurs in an area of normal mucosa. Subsequent dysplastic and ultimately carcinomatous change then occurs.
Diffuse type	Single cell changes occur in the mucus neck of the gastric glands, proliferation of these cells out of the crypts then allows invasion into the lamina propria.

Which other types have been identified?

Lymphoma, squamous cell carcinoma, adenoacanthoma, carcinoid, leiomyosarcoma.

What is the Borrmann classification system for gastric cancer?

This defines the macroscopic appearance of the lesion:

Type 1	Well circumscribed, polypoid lesion,
Type II	Fungating polypoid lesion (central infiltration),
Type III	Ulcerated with infiltrative margins,
Type IV	Linitis plastica (infiltrating).

Which presenting clinical features may be associated with gastric cancer?

Presenting features are usually vague, which is why gastric cancer is usually diagnosed at a late stage. These include: symptoms of gastro-oesophageal reflux, abdominal fullness or early satiety, belching and rarely nausea, vomiting or GI bleeding. Dysphagia may be present in patients with proximal tumours or lesions at the gastro-oesophageal junction. Late features also include weight loss, anaemia, abdominal pain or mass, and features of hepatic or intraperitoneal metastases.

Which para-neoplastic conditions may be associated with gastric cancer?

- Acanthosis nigricans,
- Dermatomyositis.

Briefly describe the key diagnostic investigations you may require in a patient in whom you suspect gastric cancer

Upper GI endoscopy and biopsy –– Can provide a histological diagnosis and is the 'gold standard' diagnostic test. Endoscopy does not, however, give functional information on motility or extrinsic compression.

Double contrast barium swallow –– Allows direct visualization of the stomach mucosa and may show a reduction in distensibility in cases of diffuse infiltrative malignancy. Although unable to differentiate clearly between benign and malignant lesions, associated obstruction or extrinsic compression by lesions outside the GI tract may be visible.

CT (chest or abdomen/pelvis) –– To establish extent of both local and metastatic spread and allow formal staging of the disease.

Briefly outline the primary tumour staging of gastric cancer

T0   No evidence of primary,

Tis   Intraepithelial carcinoma *in situ*; does not invade the lamina propria,

T1   Invades the lamina propria or submucosa,

T2   Invades the muscularis propria,

T3   Invades the serosa without local invasion of surrounding structures,

T4   Direct local invasion.

Which regional lymph nodes are involved in local nodal spread of gastric cancer?

The peri-gastric nodes and the nodes along the left gastric, common hepatic, splenic and coeliac arteries. At least 15 lymph nodes should be examined, to allow accurate nodal staging.

What is the role of laparoscopic staging in gastric cancer?

The goal of laparoscopic staging is to provide accurate staging and assessment, visualizing hepatic and peritoneal deposits below the resolution of non-invasive imaging and allowing assessment of the extent of the primary tumour. This facilitates patient selection not only for surgery but also for neo-adjuvant treatment and chemotherapy alone in irresectable disease.

Following port insertion, 200 ml of normal saline is instilled into the peritoneal cavity, specimens are then aspirated from the pelvis, subhepatic space and left upper quadrant, and sent for cytology. The abdominal structures, peri-gastric nodes, visceral and parietal peritoneum are then inspected systematically for evidence of metastatic disease. Lymph node biopsies are not routinely taken during laparoscopic staging.

What are the procedure specific complications of total gastrectomy?

Early –– Anastomotic leak, pancreatitis, cholecystitis, haemorrhage, infection.

Late –– Dumping syndrome, vitamin B12 deficiency (lack of intrinsic factor normally produced by the stomach), metabolic bone disease, and recurrence of malignancy.

What is dumping syndrome?

Loss of the reservoir function of the stomach (e.g., following gastrectomy) results in the rapid transit of highly osmotically active substances into the duodenum following meals and may cause 'dumping syndrome'.

Early dumping –– Approximately 30–60 minutes following a meal, rapid transit of the hyper-osmolar gastric contents into the small bowel results in a fluid shift from the intravascular compartment to the gastric lumen and small bowel distension. Clinically, this presents as colicky abdominal pain, diarrhoea and vasomotor symptoms, such as tachycardia and postural hypotension. It is likely that exaggerated production of gut hormones also contributes to 'early dumping' through a variety of mechanisms, ultimately enhancing sympathetic outflow.

Late dumping –– This occurs 1–3 hours following meals. Rapid transit of carbohydrate into the small bowel results in sudden absorption of high levels of glucose and compensatory hyper-insulinaemia, resulting in subsequent hypoglycaemia.

Oesophageal and gastric malignancy

What are the commonest histological types of oesophageal cancer?

- Squamous cell carcinoma,
- Adenocarcinoma.

Which key aetiological factors are associated with the development of oesophageal cancer?

Smoking	Associated with the development of both adenocarcinoma and squamous cell carcinoma,
Alcohol consumption	May increase the risk of squamous cell carcinoma,
Gastro-oesophageal reflux disease	Chronic GORD may lead to the development of squamous to columnar metaplasia in the distal oesophagus (Barrett's oesophagus), which may develop dysplastic changes and in turn carcinoma *in situ* or invasive adenocarcinoma,
Obesity	Association with adenocarcinoma of the oesophagus.

Note: *H. pylori* infection is associated with a reduction in the risk of adenocarcinoma of the oesophagus.

How may oesophageal cancer present?

1. Progressive dysphagia,
2. Odynophagia,
3. Vomiting: typically undigested food,
4. Weight loss,
5. Hoarseness (L recurrent laryngeal nerve involvement),
6. Cough (potential trachea-oesophageal fistula),
7. Metastatic disease: palpable lymph nodes, ascites, bone pain.

The diagnosis is ultimately made on upper GI endoscopy and histological assessment of biopsy specimens. CT staging and occasionally positron emission tomography (PET) imaging are used in the assessment of disseminated disease.

List the potential surgical approaches to oesophagectomy

Ivor–Lewis oesophagectomy –– May be performed as either a single or a staged procedure. The approach is via an upper midline laparotomy and right posterolateral thoracotomy. The proximal stomach and distal oesophagus are mobilized with division of the left gastric artery and vein. The accompanying lymph nodes are also resected. At this stage, a pyloroplasty is usually performed to aid gastric emptying. The stomach is then divided and tubularized and the gastric conduit passed through the diaphragmatic hiatus (which may need to be enlarged) into the posterior mediastinum. The abdomen is then closed and the patient is placed in left lateral decubitus position for the right posterolateral thoracotomy. The azygous vein is divided. The thoracic duct is preserved and large branches clipped to prevent chylothorax. The oesophago-gastric specimen and tubularized stomach are pulled up into the chest and the specimen resected with accompanying lymph nodes. A stapled or hand-sewn anastomosis may then be performed. A nasogastric tube, two chest drains and surgical drains are placed prior to closure.

McKeown oesophagectomy −− Performed via a three-incision approach, this is a modification of the Ivor–Lewis oesophagectomy. This procedure begins with the right posterolateral thoracotomy and oesophageal mobilization. An upper midline laparotomy is then performed; the stomach is mobilized and a gastric tube created. Finally, a low collar or anterior sternocleidomastoid incision is made in the left neck to allow the oesophago-gastric specimen to be pulled up into the neck. Here, the specimen is resected and either a stapled or hand-sewn anastomosis is performed. The benefit of this procedure is that it allows a wider resection margin with complete resection of tumours of the upper and middle third of the oesophagus.

Trans-hiatal oesophagectomy −− This approach avoids the need for a thoracotomy incision. It begins with an upper midline laparotomy incision with mobilization of the stomach and pyloroplasty. The distal oesophagus is then mobilized manually through the diaphragmatic hiatus via blunt dissection. An incision along the anterior sternocleidomastoid is then performed and dissection made down to the level of the prevertebral fascia. The tracheo-esophageal groove is then dissected, mobilizing the oesophagus in the superior mediastinum. Blunt dissection is then performed with the right hand placed through the abdominal incision into the oesophageal hiatus and the left hand through the cervical incision until the surgeon's fingers meet in the middle. The oesophagus is then divided and pulled into the abdomen and the stomach tubularized. The gastric conduit is then passed through the diaphragmatic hiatus and the anastomosis performed in the neck. The benefit of this approach is that performing the anastomosis within the neck reduces intrathoracic leaks and mediastinitis.

Left thoraco-abdominal oesophagectomy −− This approach is performed using a left thoraco-abdominal incision. It is particularly useful for tumours of the distal third of the oesophagus or the gastro-oesophageal junction, as it provides excellent exposure of this region. After entering the chest, a circumferential incision is made along the edge of the diaphragm, the mediastinal pleura incised and the oesophagus mobilized. The proximal oesophagus is divided and the stomach delivered through the oesophageal hiatus. The anastomosis is performed within the chest. A pyloroplasty may then be performed prior to repair of the diaphragm and closure with drain placement.

Chapter

12

The liver, biliary tree and pancreas

Gallstone disease

Briefly explain the processes involved in the formation and excretion of bilirubin

Bilirubin is produced in the spleen and reticuloendothelial system as the terminal product of haem catabolism. Unconjugated bilirubin is transported from the spleen in the blood bound to plasma albumin. In the liver, bilirubin is released from albumin and taken up by hepatocytes where conjugation (glucuronidation) occurs by the action of UDP glucuronyl transferase. Bilirubin is then released into the gut where deconjugation and conversion to urobilinogen occurs by the action of gut bacteria. Urobilinogen (water-soluble) is partially reabsorbed by the gut into the portal system (enterohepatic circulation), whilst the remainder is oxidized in the colon to produce stercobilinogen, the brown faecal pigment. Traces of urobilinogen reach the systemic circulation and are excreted in the urine.

List the commonest types of gallstone

Cholesterol stones (~80%) –– These are often formed as large, solitary gallstones and are made up of cholesterol monohydrate crystals. These form when the cholesterol concentration of bile exceeds the ability of bile salts to dissolve cholesterol and lectin. This may occur either as a result of supersaturation of the bile with cholesterol or as a result of bile salt deficiency.

Black pigment stones (~15–20%) –– These are formed from calcium bilirubinate and inorganic calcium salts, including calcium phosphate and calcium carbonate, these are usually small and multiple. They commonly form in conditions, such as chronic haemolysis or alcoholic liver disease, where there is high haem turnover and a higher concentration of unconjugated bilirubin in the bile. The black colour occurs because of repeated oxidation of bilirubin.

Brown pigment stones (<1% in the UK and USA, up to 20% in China or Taiwan, 2-3% in Japan) –– These form from calcium bilirubinate and calcium palmitate or stearate (fatty acids) and mucin. They have a greasy, soft consistency and may be associated with biliary infection or liver fluke (or other parasitic) infestation. Unlike other forms of gallstone, which develop in the gallbladder (GB), brown pigment stones develop in the ducts, behind an area of stricture or inflammation.

Mixed cholesterol and pigment stones –– These form from the accumulation of calcium salts such as calcium bilirubinate with cholesterol stones.

What are the clinical features of biliary colic?

Intermittent impaction of gallstones within the cystic duct may cause pain during gallbladder contraction, resulting in biliary colic. Right upper quadrant pain with associated nausea and vomiting are common presenting features. Pain may last up to 6–12 hours with each episode of colic. Fever and rigors suggest cholecystitis or pancreatitis. Painless jaundice with significant associated weight loss carries a very high suspicion of malignancy (most commonly adenocarcinoma of the head of pancreas).

What is Charcot's triad?

This is the triad of right upper quadrant pain, jaundice and pyrexia. It is characteristic of ascending cholangitis.

What level does serum bilirubin commonly reach before jaundice is clinically visible?

Approximately 50 μmol/l.

Which investigations are important in the diagnosis of biliary disease?

Blood tests

Full blood count	Anaemia secondary to haemolysis or malignancy.
Liver function	Predominantly raised ALP implies a posthepatic, obstructive pattern of jaundice whereas predominantly raised transaminases imply a hepatic cause.
Conjugated and unconjugated bilirubin	Unconjugated bilirubinaemia implies a prehepatic cause; conjugated bilirubinaemia implies a hepatic or posthepatic cause.
Clotting	Clotting dysfunction implies a functional impairment of hepatic function.

Imaging

Ultrasound	Gallstones within the gallbladder produce an acoustic shadow. Peri-cholecystic fluid and wall thickening may indicate acute cholecystitis and although USS is unreliable at assessing stones within the ducts, >8 mm dilatation of the common bile duct is pathological. Assessment of the liver and intrahepatic ducts is also performed.
CT	Is less sensitive than USS in detecting gallstones although is used where there is a suspicion of malignancy.
Magnetic resonance cholangio-pancreatography (MRCP)	Used as a diagnostic test and is highly sensitive in detecting cholelithiasis both within the GB and the ducts.
Endoscopic retrograde cholangio-pancreatogram (ERCP)	After the endoscope is passed into the duodenum, the ampulla of Vater is cannulated and contrast is injected into the biliary tree. Fluoroscopy is performed and assessment made for filling defects within the ducts. If the presence of gallstones is confirmed, endoscopic extraction and sphincterotomy may be performed, thus making ERCP both a diagnostic and therapeutic technique.

Describe the indications for cholecystectomy

1. Symptomatic cholelithiasis (either single or recurrent episodes of biliary colic with proven gallstone disease),

2. Biliary dyskinesia,

3. Porcelain gallbladder identified on imaging (increased risk of cholangiocarcinoma),

4. Acute cholecystitis,

5. Complications related to common bile duct stones, including pancreatitis.

Note: There is continued debate over the indications for delayed vs. acute cholecystectomy in acute cholecystitis. Early cholecystectomy should usually be performed within 24 hours of diagnosis and delayed scheduled at 6–8 weeks following the last exacerbation.

Briefly describe the technique of laparoscopic cholecystectomy

After insertion of the umbilical port (12 mm) and creation of pneumoperitoneum, a further three ports are inserted (two right and one left hypochondrial). An initial laparoscopy is performed to exclude any other gross abdominal pathology. To expose Calot's triangle, the fundus of the gallbladder is grasped and lifted towards the right lobe of the liver. The triangular fold of peritoneum (cystic pedicle) containing the cystic duct (anterior) and artery (postero-superiorly), the cystic node is identified. The entry of the cystic duct into the right side of the common bile duct is identified, to confirm the anatomy. The cystic duct and artery are clipped and ligated and the gallbladder can then be dissected free from the liver bed. The gallbladder is then extracted through the umbilical port, the liver bed examined and haemostasis ensured. Wash-out of the subhepatic and right parahepatic spaces is performed and after a final general examination to exclude any inadvertent damage during laparoscopy, the ports are removed under direct vision. A drain may be left *in situ* in the gallbladder bed if indicated.

What are the specific complications associated with this procedure?

Immediate –– Common bile duct injury, bile leak, haemorrhage, bile leak, spillage of gallstones, bowel injury.

Early –– Retained stone in CBD, abscess formation, bleeding, pancreatitis.

Late –– Adhesions, gallstone abscess.

How may biliary leaks be classified?

Many systems exist to classify bile duct injuries. One example is the Strasberg classification:

Type A Leak from a minor duct still in continuity with the common bile duct. This is commonly caused by a leak from either an accessory duct (e.g., duct of Luschka) or a cystic duct stump.

Type B Occlusion of part of the biliary tree, usually due to injury to an aberrant right hepatic duct.

Type C Leak from duct not in communication with the common bile duct (usually due to transection of an aberrant right hepatic duct, which has not been ligated).

Type D Lateral injury to any major extrahepatic bile duct (the common hepatic duct, common bile duct or extrahepatic portions of the right or left hepatic ducts). The intra-hepatic ducts remain intact.

Type E Circumferential injury to the extrahepatic bile duct separating the liver from its drainage into the biliary tree. This may be due to either transection or stricturing.

Gallbladder malignancy

Is the presence of gallstones associated with the development of gallbladder (GB) malignancy?

Yes. Whilst causality is difficult to demonstrate, gallstones are found in up to 75–90% of cases of gallbladder malignancy and the risk has been shown to increase with gallstone size. Porcelain gallbladder has also been associated with malignancy, although the incidence of this is variable within the literature.

What is the most common histological subtype of gallbladder cancer?

Approximately 90% of gallbladder malignancies are adenocarcinoma. Other histological types include squamous cell carcinoma, sarcoma, adenosquamous, carcinoid, lymphoma and metastatic cancers. Adenomatous polyps may also occur within the gallbladder and carry malignant potential.

What are the presenting features of gallbladder malignancy?

Gallbladder malignancies are commonly asymptomatic until the late stages, giving rise to a poor five-year survival rate of approximately 5%. Features such as weight loss, right upper quadrant (RUQ) mass or painless jaundice are suggestive of malignancy. Patients presenting with symptoms of acute cholecystitis may be diagnosed at an earlier stage, improving prognosis. Approximately two-thirds of gallbladder malignancies are 'incidental' findings at cholecystectomy.

Which tumour markers may be raised in gallbladder cancer?

CEA (carcinoembryonic antigen) and CA19–9 (carbohydrate antigen 19–9)

Briefly describe the staging of gallbladder cancer

This is based on the TNM staging system and has been developed by the International Union Against Cancer (UICC) and the American Joint Committee on Cancer (AJCC):

Stage 0 (Tis N0 M0)	Carcinoma *in situ*,
Stage IA (T1 N0 M0)	Invades the lamina propria or muscle layer,
Stage IB (T2 N0 M0)	Invasion into peri-muscular connective tissue,
Stage IIA (T3 N0 M0)	Invades the serosa or directly invades the liver or one other organ,
Stage IIB (T1–3 N1 M0)	Invasion as described above with regional lymph node metastasis,
Stage III (T4 N0+ M0)	Invades the portal vein, common hepatic artery or more than one extrahepatic organ,

Stage IV (T1–4 N0+ M1)   Distant metastases, including nodal metastases to the pancreatic body and tail.

What are the surgical options available for the management of gallbladder malignancy?

The management of these patients should be discussed within a multidisciplinary team both in cases where resection is possible and in those where it is unlikely to confer benefit. Surgical options include:

1. Simple cholecystectomy in Tis, T1A and T1B with negative resection margins,
2. Radical cholecystectomy (GB resection plus 2 cm margin of GB bed plus LN dissection from the hepatoduodenal ligament behind D2, the head of the pancreas and coeliac axis),
3. Radical cholecystectomy plus segmental or lobar liver resection,
4. Radical cholecystectomy plus para-aortic LN dissection,
5. Radical cholecystectomy plus bile duct resection or pancreaticoduodenectomy.

Pancreatitis

What are the two most common causes of acute pancreatitis?

- Gallstones (approximately 45% worldwide),
- Alcohol (approximately 35%).

Approximately 20% of cases are idiopathic with no identifiable cause established.

List the less common causes of acute pancreatitis

- Drugs: steroids, NSAIDs, frusemide, sulphonamides, azathioprine,
- Autoimmune: SLE or panarteritis nodosa, associated with elevated IgG4 subtype,
- Hypercalcaemia: thought to be due to calcium deposition in the pancreatic duct and calcium activation of trypsinogen,
- Trauma,
- Iatrogenic: following ERCP or abdominal surgery,
- Sphincter of Oddi dysfunction, resulting in transient pancreatic duct obstruction (may occur following cholecystectomy),
- Anatomical variations, such as pancreas divisum,
- Pancreatic ischaemia secondary to vascular pathology,
- Toxins.

What are the common presenting clinical features of acute pancreatitis?

- Pain: acute, severe epigastric pain radiating to the back, relieved on sitting forwards,
- Vomiting,
- Features of a systemic inflammatory response: tachycardia, tachypnoea, pyrexia or low temperature, hypotension.

Clinical signs include:

Grey-Turner's sign	Haemorrhage tracking from the anterior pararenal space, between the leaves of posterior renal fascia to the lateral edge of quadratus lumborum.
Cullen's sign	Tracking of pancreatic enzymes to the anterior abdominal wall via the gastrohepatic and falciform ligaments.

What is the role of serum amylase in the diagnosis of acute pancreatitis?

Elevated serum amylase above three times the normal level supports the diagnosis of acute pancreatitis, but is not a predictor of severity. Serum amylase usually rises within a few hours of the onset of symptoms and returns to normal within three to five days. However, in up to 19% of patients, serum amylase may be normal on admission.

Why may serum lipase be a better diagnostic marker of acute pancreatitis?

Serum lipase levels remain elevated for longer than serum amylase, providing an advantage in those patients with a delayed presentation.

What are the modified Glasgow criteria for scoring acute pancreatitis?

- $PO_2 < 8$ kPa,
- Age > 55 years,
- Neutrophils (WCC > 15),
- Calcium < 2.0 mmol/l,
- Renal: Urea > 16 mmol/l,
- Enzymes: Lactate dehydrogenase > 600 IU/l; aspartate transaminase > 200 IU/l,
- Albumin < 32 g/dl,
- Sugar: Glucose > 10 mmol/l.

Note: The modified Glasgow criteria were designed for assessment within the first 48 hours of symptom onset and have been validated for pancreatitis due to both alcohol and gallstone disease.

Which other scoring systems are frequently used?

Many scoring systems are available. The most commonly used are Ranson and APACHE-II (Acute Physiology and Chronic Health Evaluation-II).

List the Ranson criteria in the scoring of acute (non-gallstone) pancreatitis

Ranson's criteria are applied during the first 48 h following the onset of pancreatitis. They are defined as follows:

At time of onset
- Age > 55 years,
- WCC >15 × 10^9/l,
- LDH > 600 IU/l,
- AST > 200 IU/l,
- Glucose >10 mmol/l with no previous history of diabetes.

Within the first 48 hours
- Corrected calcium < 2.0 mmol/l,
- Urea > 16mmol/l without improvement with IV fluid resuscitation,
- PO_2 < 8 kPa,
- Base deficit < −4,
- Fall in haematocrit > 10%,
- Fluid deficit > 6 l,
- Rise in serum urea nitrogen (BUN) > 5 mg/dl.

How do these criteria differ in gallstone pancreatitis?

At time of onset
- Age > 70 years,
- Glucose > 12.2 mmol/l,
- WCC > 18 × 10^9/l,
- AST > 250 IU/l,
- LDH > 400 IU/l.

Criteria after 48 hours of admission
- Fluid deficit > 4 l,
- Base deficit < −5,
- BUN rise > 2 mg/dl.

How do the Ranson criteria relate to the predicted mortality in acute pancreatitis?

Mortality is predicted based on the number of positive criteria:

    0–2 <5% mortality,

    3–4 20% mortality,

5–6 40% mortality,

7–8 100% mortality.

What is the Atlanta classification system?

This classification system was originally defined in 1992 and forms the basis of the British Society of Gastroenterology (BSG) guidelines in the assessment of acute pancreatitis. Severity scoring is based on the Ranson or APACHE-II scores. Organ failure and systemic complications are considered, as well as local complications, such as fluid collection, pseudocyst, pancreatic abscess and necrosis.

Which features are associated with a severe attack of acute pancreatitis?

The UK guidelines on acute pancreatitis state that the following features suggest an acute, severe episode of pancreatitis:

Initial assessment –– Clinical impression of severity; body mass index > 30; pleural effusion on chest radiograph; APACHE-II score $\geq$ 8.

24 after admission –– Clinical impression of severity; APACHE-II score $\geq$ 8; Glasgow score $\geq$ 3; persisting organ failure, especially if multiple, C-reactive protein $\geq$ 150 mg/l.

48 after admission –– Clinical impression of severity; Glasgow score $\geq$ 3; C-reactive protein $\geq$ 150 mg/l; persisting organ failure for 48 hrs; multiple or progressive organ failure.

Describe the key points in the management of acute pancreatitis

The current UK guidelines advise that all patients with acute pancreatitis should be treated aggressively until disease severity has been established. Key points include:

1. Oxygen supplementation: continuous monitoring and maintenance of pulse oximetry saturations >95%.

2. Adequate prompt fluid resuscitation has been shown to reduce systemic complications and the development of organ failure. Aim to maintain minimum urine output at 0.5 ml/(kg h).

3. Patients with moderate to severe disease should be managed in an HDU/ITU environment and continuous assessment of organ function made with invasive monitoring where necessary (e.g., CVP, arterial lines).

4. Early initiation of nutrition is important to maintain a positive nitrogen balance. Parenteral nutrition may be necessary; however, the enteral route may be used where tolerated.

5. Treatment of the underlying cause: e.g., in severe acute gallstone pancreatitis. Urgent therapeutic ERCP and sphincterotomy within the first 72 hours may be required.

6. Surgical management: infected necrotic pancreatitis may require necrosectomy. Closure of the abdomen may not be possible following this procedure and the abdomen may be packed or closed over drains, through which irrigation may be performed.

What is the role of antibiotic therapy in the treatment of acute pancreatitis?

There is currently no consensus on the use of prophylactic antibiotics, the type of agent or the duration of therapy in the management of acute pancreatitis. It is also unlikely that antibiotic prophylaxis has an effect on outcomes in patients without necrotic pancreatitis. It is therefore not routine to prescribe antibiotic prophylaxis in patients with mild to moderate pancreatitis where no focal infection has been identified. Where antibiotic prophylaxis is decided upon, UK guidelines suggest that it should be limited to 7–14 days.

What are the common complications of acute pancreatitis?

Local complications:
1. Peri-pancreatic fluid collection,
2. Pancreatic or peri-pancreatic abscess,
3. Pseudocyst formation,
4. Pancreatic necrosis.

Systemic complications:
1. Coagulopathy,
2. Renal failure (thought to be due to a combination of toxic injury from vasoactive peptides and inflammatory mediators and decreased renal blood flow secondary to hypovolaemia),
3. Hypocalcaemia (due to a combination of saponification of calcium salts with free fatty acids, glucagon stimulated calcitonin release and decreased parathyroid hormone secretion),
4. Hyperglycaemia (failure of endocrine function of the pancreas),
5. Respiratory failure (atelectasis, pneumonitis, pleural effusions and ultimately adult respiratory distress syndrome),
6. Hypovolaemia and systemic shock.

What is chronic pancreatitis?

This is chronic and irreversible inflammation, leading to fibrosis and calcification of the pancreas. There is a failure of both endocrine and exocrine function of the gland, resulting in malabsorption and diabetes mellitus.

Which aetiological factors are associated with its development?

1. Environmental factors: alcohol and smoking,

2. Cystic fibrosis,

3. Ductal obstruction: e.g., due to anatomical variations, abdominal trauma, stone disease or malignancy,

4. Autoimmune pancreatitis, associated with primary sclerosing cholangitis, Sjogren's syndrome and primary biliary cirrhosis,

5. Idiopathic.

What are the common histological changes in chronic pancreatitis?

Chronic pancreatitis is characterized by destruction and loss of acinar cells, interlobular fibrosis, cellular infiltration, ductal protein plugs, dilation and lithiasis. In addition, ductal epithelial hyperplasia or metaplasia may be present.

What are the key presenting features of chronic pancreatitis?

Chronic pancreatitis usually presents with one or a combination of the following:

- Central abdominal pain (epigastric) with intermittent flare-ups similar in nature to the pain of acute pancreatitis. Pain may improve over time, as with progressive pancreatic dysfunction and calcification.

- Failure of exocrine function: malabsorption resulting in steatorrhoea, fat soluble vitamin (A, D, E, K, B12) deficiency and weight loss.

- Failure of endocrine function: loss of β-cell secretory function and impairment of β-cell responsiveness leads to diabetes mellitus, which may be insulin dependent. Loss of α-cell function also results in impaired glucagon secretion, contributing to the increased susceptibility to profound hypoglycaemia in these patients.

Which investigations may be useful in the diagnosis of chronic pancreatitis?

Faecal tests –– Faecal chymotrypsin and human pancreatic elastase-1 may be useful in confirming the diagnosis in late stage pancreatitis but are not quantitative or able to detect early disease.

Duodenal or pancreatic duct aspirates –– Endoscopic sampling of duodenal or pancreatic duct fluid allows the detection of pancreatic bicarbonate, lipase, amylase and protease. This is sensitive even in early disease.

Abdominal X-ray –– This shows pancreatic calcification in 30% of patients with chronic pancreatitis.

CT scanning –– Whilst useful in advanced pancreatitis and in diagnosis of complications of pancreatitis and planning intervention, CT does not clearly depict early disease.

ERCP –– This gives an accurate visualization of the pancreatic duct and branches, and is the 'gold standard' in diagnosing chronic pancreatitis. ERCP gives little information on the pancreatic parenchyma.

MRCP –– This shows the pancreatic parenchyma, surrounding tissues and ductal structure.

Endoscopic ultrasound (EUS) –– This is both sensitive and specific, and allows for visualization of ductal stones. It may also be combined with fine needle aspiration or tru-cut biopsy to provide a histological diagnosis.

What are the key features in the management of chronic pancreatitis?

Secondary prevention –– Alcohol avoidance, smoking cessation.

Pain control –– Analgesic control in accordance with the World Health Organization (WHO) pain ladder is initially implemented. Opiates are often required. Amitriptyline may potentiate the effects of opiates and improve neuropathic pain. If conventional analgesics fail, coeliac plexus block may improve symptoms. Subcutaneous octreotide is used to reduce pancreatic exocrine secretion and may improve pain in approximately 50%.

Vitamins and antioxidant therapy –– These have been shown to reduce pain, analgesic requirement and hospitalization in some patients; however efficacy may be as low as 10–15%.

Replacement of exocrine function –– Either enteric-coated pancreatic enzymes (e.g., Creon – pancrelipase delayed release capsules) or uncoated in combination with acid suppression.

Replacement of endocrine function –– Insulin replacement therapy.

Relief of ductal obstruction –– In calcific pancreatitis, either extracorporeal shock wave lithotripsy (ESWL) or ERCP with removal of ductal stones. ERCP with sphincterotomy or stenting of the pancreatic duct may improve pain and relieve obstruction.

Surgical treatment –– Total pancreatectomy with autologous islet cell transplantation.

Pancreatic malignancy

What is the incidence of pancreatic cancer worldwide?

Approximately 8–12 cases per 100 000. Pancreatic cancer is the fifth commonest cause of cancer death and the eleventh commonest cancer in the UK.

Which predisposing aetiological factors have been identified to increase the risk of pancreatic cancer?

1. Smoking,
2. Race: African Americans,
3. Inherited syndromes (multiple endocrine neoplasia (MEN-1), colonic polyposis syndromes, (hereditary non-polyposis colorectal cancer, familial adenomatous polyposis), Von Hippel Lindau),
4. Chronic pancreatitis: alcoholic and familial.

What proportion of pancreatic cancers have distant metastases (stage IV) at the time of diagnosis?

40–50%.

What are the common sites of development of pancreatic cancers?

Approximately 95% of pancreatic cancers originate from the exocrine pancreas, 75% occur in the head or neck of the pancreas, 15–20% occur in the body and 5–10% occur in the tail.

What is the commonest histological type of pancreatic cancer?

Adenocarcinoma of the ductal epithelium (80%).

Which other, less common, exocrine tumours are known to occur?

Solid –– Primary pancreatic lymphoma, giant cell carcinoma, adenosquamous carcinoma, microglandular adenocarcinoma, mucinous carcinoma, islet cell tumours (e.g., insulinomas, glucagonomas and gastrinoma).

Cystic (5%) –– Acinar cystadenocarcinoma, cystadenocarcinoma, papillary cystic carcinoma.

What are the common sites of metastases in pancreatic cancer?

Spread is initially to the regional lymph nodes then to the liver and surrounding viscera, such as the duodenum, stomach and colon. Lung and skin metastases may rarely occur.

Which genetic mutations have been associated with pancreatic cancer?

Mutations in the KRAS2; CDKN2; p53 and Smad4 have been identified. An association has also been identified in families with BRCA-1 and BRCA-2 mutations.

Which tumour marker is particularly useful in the diagnosis of pancreatic cancer?

CA19–9. CA19–9 is elevated in 75–85% of patients with pancreatic cancer and is useful in diagnosis, staging, follow-up and response to therapy. However, it is not sufficiently sensitive in early disease to be used as a screening tool.

Which other tumour markers may be useful?

Carcinoembryonic antigen (CEA) is raised in 40–45% of patients with pancreatic cancer. However, it is not sensitive or specific to pancreatic cancer and may be raised by many other benign and malignant conditions.

Briefly outline the differences between T1 and T4 lesions in the TNM staging system for pancreatic cancer

T1	Tumour is limited to the pancreas and is 2 cm or smaller,
T2	Tumour is limited to the pancreas but is larger than 2 cm,
T3	Tumour extension beyond the pancreas (e.g., duodenum, bile duct, portal or superior mesenteric vein) but not involving the coeliac axis or superior mesenteric artery,
T4	Tumour involves the coeliac axis or superior mesenteric arteries.

Which surgical options are available in the management of pancreatic cancer?

Whipple's procedure (pancreaticoduodenectomy) –– This procedure involves resection of the pancreatic head, duodenum, proximal jejunum, common bile duct, cholecystectomy and distal gastrectomy. The pancreatic duct is anastamosed to the jejunum and en bloc resection of the regional lymph nodes is also performed. More recently, pylorus-sparing pancreaticoduodenectomy has been shown to be equally as effective with equivalent morbidity and long-term outcomes, whilst preserving some gastrointestinal function. Potential disadvantages to the pylorus-sparing approach include delayed gastric emptying and inadequate lymph node resection.

Distal pancreatectomy –– This is performed to treat tumours of the body and tail of the pancreas. The distal pancreas is isolated and usually divided in the plane between the superior mesenteric vein and the pancreatic vein. To prevent pancreatic leakage, the distal pancreatic duct is ligated and the stump oversewn.

Total pancreatectomy –– Used for treatment of tumours of the neck of the pancreas, or where there is evidence of multicentric disease. Resection involves the entire pancreas and includes duodenectomy, which may be pylorus sparing. The short gastric vessels and gastrosplenic ligaments are divided and total splenectomy is performed. The accompanying lymph node (LN) dissection involves the peri-pancreatic nodes, the lymph node along the coeliac axis, hepatic artery, splenic artery, SMA/SMV, portal vein, the retroduodenal and retropancreatic portion of the aorta and vena cava, and the common bile duct.

What are the key procedure-specific complications associated with Whipple's procedure?

1. Pancreatic anastomotic leak, resulting in leakage of pancreatic protease and lipase, which may cause inflammation and necrosis of the surrounding tissue,

2. Pancreatic fistula formation, which usually occurs as a result of pancreatic anastomotic leak,

3. Biliary anastomotic leak,

4. Peri-anastamotic collection,

5. Delayed gastric emptying, in particular associated with pylorus-sparing procedures.

The spleen: splenic trauma and splenectomy

What proportion of traumatic blunt splenic injuries are successfully treated conservatively?

Around 90%.

Which diagnostic modalities are useful in the assessment of the patient following blunt abdominal trauma?

Focused assessment for sonography in trauma (FAST) –– This includes examination of the peri-splenic region, Morrison's pouch, subxiphoid pericardial view, suprapubic region and examination of pleura for haemothoraces.

Diagnostic peritoneal lavage (DPL) –– See below.

CT with contrast –– This is the gold standard for the assessment of traumatic intra-abdominal injury. Grading of splenic injury is based on CT images. It may also be used in the quantification of intra-abdominal injury in the presence of a positive FAST or DPL.

Angiography –– This allows assessment of the site of active bleeding and intervention in the form of embolization. This is usually performed either in an attempt to avoid surgical intervention where there is contrast blush or extravasation on CT, or in the haemodynamically stable patient at high risk of re-bleeding (i.e., treatment of potential pseudo-aneurysm).

Briefly describe the procedure of DPL

DPL is performed by either an open or a Seldinger technique in the infra-umbilical position. Prior to DPL, an NG tube and urinary catheter should be placed to decompress the stomach and bladder. Once the peritoneal cavity is entered, the DPL catheter is inserted and any peritoneal fluid is aspirated. Aspiration of >10 ml of blood at this stage is considered a positive result. If this is not the case, the DPL catheter is connected to 1 litre of warmed Hartmann's solution and this is infused into the peritoneal cavity. Once the bag is almost empty, it is placed on the floor and the contents are allowed to flow back into it. A minimum of 300 ml fluid return is required for analysis. The fluid is then sent for red and white blood cell counts, gram stain and gross examination for bilious or enteric content.

What is considered as a positive result and an indication for laparotomy?

1. >10 ml blood aspirated on initial entry into the peritoneal cavity,
2. WCC > 500 per mm^3,
3. RBC > 100 000 per mm^3,
4. The presence of enteric contents.

What are the benefits of FAST over DPL?

1. FAST allows accurate diagnosis of haemoperitoneum by a non-invasive technique. Examination of the pericardium and pleura may also be performed.
2. It can be performed quickly and integrated into the primary or secondary survey.
3. It avoids the complications of DPL.

Describe the grading system used in traumatic splenic injury

This is in accordance with the American Association for the Surgery of Trauma (AAST 1994) grading system:

Grade I	Subcapsular haematoma <10% surface area. Capsular lesion <1 cm depth.
Grade II	Subcapsular haematoma 10–50% surface area. Capsular lesion 1–3 cm depth. Intra-parenchymal haematoma <5 cm diameter.
Grade III	Subcapsular haematoma >50% surface area. Capsular lesion >3 cm depth. Intra-parenchymal haematoma >5 cm diameter.
Grade IV	Laceration involving the hilar vessels producing devascularization of >25% of the spleen.
Grade V	Complete splenic fracture. Hilar vascular injury with complete splenic devascularization.

What are the indications for operative intervention in splenic trauma?

1. Haemodynamic instability with failure of fluid resuscitation and non-operative management,
2. Active bleeding as evidenced by contrast extravasation where embolization is not available and where the patient develops signs of haemodynamic disturbance,
3. High-grade injury.

Briefly describe the key operative steps in splenectomy for splenic trauma

The patient is placed in a supine position and a midline laparotomy incision is made. Once the peritoneal cavity has been entered, suction is required to improve visualization of the operative field. The spleen must first be mobilized to the midline for assessment of the extent of injury and potential repair. The surgeon places a hand into the left upper quadrant over the convex surface of the spleen. Any adhesions and the lienorenal and splenophrenic ligaments need to be divided, in order to bring the spleen (and the tail of the pancreas) into the midline. Once the spleen is mobilized, the vascular pedicle is pinched or clamped to occlude the short gastric vessels (within the gastrosplenic ligament) and the splenic hilar vessels (splenic artery and vein); this provides haemostasis. Once haemostasis is achieved, the spleen can be inspected and the potential for repair assessed. For complete splenectomy, the splenic hilar vessels are clamped and divided as close to the spleen as possible, to avoid injury to the tail of the pancreas. The gastrosplenic ligament (containing the short gastric vessels) is also clamped and divided, taking care not to damage the greater curve of the stomach. Finally, the splenocolic ligament is clamped and divided, and the spleen can be removed. Once the spleen is removed, the previously clamped vessels are ligated and wash-out of the splenic fossa and peritoneal cavity performed. The tail of the pancreas and greater curve of the stomach are then assessed for any iatrogenic injury. Drains may then be placed prior to closure if there is concern over the tail of the pancreas.

What are the early complications of total splenectomy?

- Bleeding,
- Acute gastric distension,
- Gastric necrosis,
- Pancreatic fistula,
- Pancreatitis,
- Subphrenic abscess.

What are the late complications of total splenectomy?

Overwhelming postsplenectomy infection (OPSI) –– In particular, due to encapsulated organisms, such as *S. pneumoniae*, *N. meningitidis* and *H. influenzae* type B. The risk is highest in the first two years after splenectomy. Prophylactic antibiotics and vaccination against encapsulated bacteria (Pneumovax, HibTITER, *Neisseria meningitidis* group A, C, Y, W-135) is advised in all patients.

Thrombosis –– Portal vein thrombosis and DVT are both increased following splenectomy due to thrombocytosis.

Chapter

14

The large bowel

Diverticular disease

Define what is meant by diverticular disease

Diverticular disease is herniation of mucosa through the muscularis of the colonic wall. It usually occurs at the site of relative weakness where mesenteric blood vessels pass between the taeniae coli through the colonic muscle wall.

What is the difference between a true and false diverticulum?

A true diverticulum contains all layers of the wall of the viscus (e.g., Meckel's diverticulum). A false diverticulum involves only some layers (e.g., colonic diverticulum).

What is the commonest site for diverticulae within the colon?

Sigmoid (95–98%). However, diverticulae may occur throughout the large and small bowel.

What is the prevalence of diverticular disease?

Diverticular disease becomes more prevalent with increasing age. It reaches approximately 60–65% at ages above 80 years.

Which aetiological factors are felt to be important in this condition?

Diverticular disease is a condition of Western civilization, although it is increasing in prevalence in Asia. A low-fibre diet, high in red meat and fat, is thought to increase intraluminal pressure, resulting in the development of diverticulae. Motility disorders and corticosteroid therapy have also been associated with this condition.

Which complications are commonly associated with diverticular disease?

1. Inflammation,
2. Perforation,
3. Abscess formation,

4. Lower gastrointestinal haemorrhage,
5. Fistulae,
6. Stricture.

How may diverticular disease present?

Presentation is usually with one of these complications. Typically, patients may complain of left-sided abdominal tenderness, which may be associated with signs of systemic sepsis or rectal bleeding. A colovesical fistula may present with pneumaturia or pyuria and faeculant vaginal discharge may represent a colovaginal tract. In the late stages, perforation will present with signs of generalized peritonitis, although these may be more insidious in early onset. Rectal bleeding is usually dark, fresh blood often with clots. It may be massive and require fluid resuscitation and significant blood transfusion.

Which investigations would you perform?

Blood tests –– FBC, inflammatory markers, clotting, group and save and cross match as necessary.

Chest X-ray (erect) and abdominal X-ray –– Look for signs of perforation (subdiaphragmatic free air, Rigler's sign) or obstruction.

CT –– This is the investigation of choice as it allows visualization of the bowel wall, assessment of peri-colic and bowel wall oedema and inflammation. It also enables identification of abscesses, perforation or fistulae. It may also clarify potential differential diagnoses and can be used for intervention (e.g., percutaneous drainage of abscesses).

Colonoscopy –– This may be useful to confirm the diagnosis of diverticular disease. In the setting of controlled colonic bleeding, colonoscopy is useful to rule out malignant causes. Specific risks associated with colonoscopy in diverticular disease include creation of false lumen and perforation.

What is the management of diverticular disease presenting as pain and systemic sepsis where there is no active bleeding?

It is important to exclude perforation in this setting. Management should be with adequate fluid rehydration and antibiotic therapy. If symptoms fail to improve, the potential for abscess formation should be considered and percutaneous drainage considered where necessary. Ultimately, surgical intervention may be required in the form of local resection and wash-out often as a staged procedure with temporary stoma formation. Surgical options include: Hartmann's procedure (local sigmoid resection with formation of end colostomy +/− mucous fistula), local resection with wash-out and primary anastomosis (with or without defunctioning stoma, depending on the level of contamination and patient's premorbid condition).

How might you classify perforation secondary to diverticulosis?

The Hinchey scoring system

Hinchey Ia   Localized peri-colic inflammation or phlegmon,

Hinchey Ib   Localized paracolic abscess,

Hinchey II   Pelvic or retrocolic abscess,

Hinchey III   Purulent peritonitis,

Hinchey IV   Faeculant peritonitis.

Hinchey I and II are acutely treated with systemic antibiotics and regular review. Hinchey II may also require percutaneous drainage. Hinchey III and IV require urgent surgical intervention.

How would you manage acute lower GI haemorrhage secondary to diverticular disease?

The initial management should be resuscitation in accordance with guidelines for adult life support and care of the critically ill patient (ALS/CCriSP). Two large-bore peripheral cannulae should be inserted and the patient given fluid and blood products as necessary. Attention should be paid to correction of clotting in the event of massive haemorrhage and subsequent transfusion. CT angiography may give information on the site of bleeding if the patient is sufficiently haemodynamically stable to undergo scanning. Active bleeding may be treated with embolization by mesenteric angiography, although in the event of haemodynamic instability and massive haemorrhage the patient should be taken to theatre as a matter of urgency. If the site of bleeding cannot be localized, subtotal colectomy may be required.

What proportion of patients experience recurrence after a first episode of diverticulitis treated medically?

Approximately one-third.

Inflammatory bowel disease: ulcerative colitis and Crohn's disease

Describe the features distinguishing ulcerative colitis (UC) from Crohn's disease

Whilst a range of factors may distinguish UC from Crohn's, the diagnosis should be based on a combination of both histological and endoscopic features and may remain unclear.

Histological

Crohn's   Multiple granulomas, deep fissures and transmural lymphoid aggregates.

UC   Inflammation is limited to the mucosa and submucosa. Crypt distortion and crypt abscesses are present with a mixed inflammatory cell infiltrate. Histological changes in Crohn's are discontinuous and may occur at several focal points, whereas in UC they are confined to the colon, are continuous and may increase in more distal parts of the colon.

Macroscopic

Crohn's   Features of *'cobblestoning'* with deep ulcers in surrounding macroscopically normal mucosa. Crohn's most commonly spares the rectum and focal areas of inflammation are seen, typically involving the ileocaecal valve and terminal ileum.

UC   UC mucosa appears friable and grossly ulcerated with vascular distortion. Pseudopolyp formation and stricturing may be seen in both UC and Crohn's; however, UC usually ends abruptly at the ileocaecal valve without terminal ileal involvement.

What is the prevalence of UC?

- UC occurs in approximately 35–100 per 100 000 of the population in the USA.
- There are two peaks in its presentation: the first occurs at age 15–25; the second at age 55–65.
- UC shows a female preponderance. The rectum is involved in 95% of cases.

How might IBD present?

Presentation is commonly with abdominal pain and associated bloody stool. Urgency of defecation may be present and stool may contain excessive mucous. Weight loss may also be evident, with features of a generalized inflammatory response and hypovolaemia in advanced stages (tachycardia, raised inflammatory markers and pyrexia).

Which autoantibody is associated with UC?

p-ANCA (anti-neutrophil cytoplasmic antibody).

Which aetiological factors are associated with UC?

Genetic   Loci on chromosomes 1, 6, 12 and 19 have been linked with a susceptibility to UC, although the genetic association is less clear than in Crohn's disease.

Smoking   Is protective against UC.

Appendectomy   Appears to be associated with a protective effect on UC.

What are the extracolonic manifestations of UC?

Opthalmological	Synovitis, episcleritis, iritis,
Dermatological	Pyoderma gangrenosum, erythema nodosum, aphthous stomatitis,
Rheumatological	Ankylosing spondylitis (HLA-B27), sacroiliitis,
Abdominal	Primary sclerosing cholangitis (PSC),
Genitourinary	Uric acid renal stones,
Haematological	Thromboembolic events.

What are the macroscopic and histological features of UC?

Macroscopic -- Evidence of generalized ulceration and inflammation throughout the colon without intervening areas of normal mucosa.

Histological -- Inflammation is limited to the mucosa and submucosa. Neutrophil infiltration is seen with the development of crypt abscesses and shortening and distortion of the crypts. The lamina propria is infiltrated with lymphoid aggregates, including plasma cells, mast cells and eosinophils.

What is the mainstay of medical management in UC?

The aim of medical management in ulcerative colitis is to improve quality of life and to induce and maintain remission.

Maintenance of remission

Immunomodulatory drugs	e.g., Azathioprine, Cyclosporin, 6-mercaptopurine (6-MP). Used as steroid-sparing or steroid-reducing agents. These drugs may also be used to induce remission in acute disease.
5-Aminosalysilic acid derivatives (5-ASAs)	e.g., Sulfasalazine. Reduce local inflammation and systemic prostaglandin synthesis.
Anti-TNFs	e.g., Infliximab.

Acute management

Corticosteroids	e.g., Hydrocortisone and Prednisolone. Use in short term induction of remission. Side effects prevent long-term usage.
Antibiotic therapy	Broad-spectrum antibiotics are often used where there is evidence of acute infection, abscess formation or perforation.
Cyclosporin A	Short-term IV infusions may be used in the acute management of steroid refractory UC.

What is the role of colonoscopic screening in UC?

Current NICE recommendations (March 2011) suggest that colonoscopic surveillance should be offered in patients with UC who have had symptoms for ten years. A baseline colonoscopy with targeted biopsies should initially be performed and the patient then categorized into low, intermediate and high risk of developing colorectal cancer. Low-risk patients are offered repeat colonoscopy at five years, intermediate-risk at three years and high-risk at one year. CT colonoscopy should be considered as a second screening tool where colonoscopy is inappropriate. Double contrast barium enema offers a third alternative.

What is the role of surgery in UC?

Acute –– Fulminant colitis refractory to maximal medical therapy, evidence of perforation, toxic megacolon (transverse colon diameter >6cm), acute obstruction secondary to stricturing disease, acute haemorrhage.

Long-term –– Prevention of malignancy, systemic complications of long-term medical therapy, recurrent episodes of colitis despite medical management.

What would be the commonest surgical procedure in the setting of acute fulminant colitis?

Subtotal colectomy and end ileostomy –– In the acute setting of fulminant colitis, this remains the safest option and offers the lowest surgical morbidity and mortality. The rectal stump is left *in situ*, and may be either exteriorized, sutured to the anterior abdominal wall, or left within the peritoneal cavity. The advantage of the first two options is a reduction in the rates of pelvic abscess formation and facilitation of future localization of the stump. Any recurrence of disease within the rectum can often be managed medically. A definitive or reconstructive procedure may then be carried out once the acute exacerbation has settled and the patient's nutritional state has been optimized.

What are the indications for elective surgery in UC?

Broadly, these include failure of maximal medical therapy or side effects of medical treatment, malignancy or high-grade dysplasia, stricturing disease and, occasionally, the presence of severe extracolonic manifestations.

Which operative options are available in the elective setting?

Pan-proctocolectomy with end ileostomy –– This resection removes the entire diseased colon and eliminates the colonic cancer risk in these patients. An end ileostomy removes the potential for functional problems with defecation frequency and urgency. In patients with proven rectal malignancy or anal sphincter dysfunction, this is often the procedure of choice. Occasionally patients may elect to have only one procedure and prefer to live with an end ileostomy rather than undergo a restorative procedure.

Subtotal colectomy and ileorectal anastomosis -- This procedure is occasionally used in patients with minimal rectal involvement or indeterminate colitis. It must be remembered that recurrence of rectal disease may occur and the risk for development of malignancy in the rectal stump is not eliminated. This procedure is now rarely performed.

Restorative proctocolectomy with ileal pouch-anal anastomosis (IPAA) -- Whilst often limited to specialist centres, this procedure is becoming more frequently the procedure of choice for UC patients. Its advantages are removal of the entire colon and rectum with a consequent reduction in malignancy risk and in problems with rectal disease recurrence; it also offers the benefit of life without a permanent stoma. However, a temporary loop ileostomy is commonly formed to cover the IPAA during the initial six weeks following the procedure. In addition, complications include anastomotic dehiscence and development of pelvic sepsis, collections and fistulae. Other disadvantages include bowel function irregularity, potential inflammation of the ileal pouch (pouchitis) and the need to continue surveillance of the anal transition zone for malignancy.

What is the prevalence of Crohn's disease?

Approximately 7 per 100 000 in the USA. Rates are highest in Europe and the USA and lowest in South Africa and Latin America.

Which other aetiological factors have been associated with Crohn's disease?

Smoking	Has been shown to up to double the risk of developing Crohn's disease.
Sex	There is a very slight female preponderance, approximately 1.2:1.
Racial	Increased in the Jewish population. Slightly increased incidence in whites.
Socioeconomic class	Crohn's is more prevalent amongst the higher socioeconomic classes.
Drugs	NSAIDs and the oral contraceptive pill have been shown to increase the risk of development of Crohn's.
Genetic	Mutations in the NOD2/CARD15 gene have been shown to confer susceptibility to Crohn's.

Which autoantibody may be associated with Crohn's disease?

Anti-*Saccharomyces cerevisiae* antibody (ASCA)

What are the key indications for surgery in Crohn's disease?

Elective or semi-elective –– Inability to obtain adequate disease control, medication side effects or progression despite maximal medical therapy often necessitates surgical intervention in Crohn's disease. Chronic progressive stricturing disease may also require surgical intervention in the semi-elective setting.

Emergency –– Complications, such as intestinal obstruction secondary to stricturing disease, may necessitate emergency resection. Peri-anal disease often requires surgical intervention for alleviation of sepsis and treatment of complex fistulae where medical management has failed. Rarely, emergency surgery may be required in the setting of acute perforation or haemorrhage.

Describe the surgical treatment of small bowel or colonic Crohn's disease

Resection –– Whilst failure of medical therapy and associated complications of Crohn's disease often necessitates resection, the most conservative safe approach should be used. The panenteric nature of this disease and likelihood of repeated exacerbations puts these patients at risk from malabsorbtive complications as a result of repeated resections. It has been reported that stapled, side-to-side anastamoses may result in lower rates of stricturing at the site of the anastamosis, although this is not universal and the calibre of bowel may favour a hand-sewn approach in some situations.

Stricturoplasty –– This is often used as an alternative to resection in an attempt to reduce the risk of 'short bowel syndrome'. Short fibrous strictures or multiple strictures in a diffuse pattern throughout the small bowel may favour stricturoplasty. Strictures within a short segment of bowel or disease recurrence at the site of previous resection contraindicate the use of this technique. The potential for malignancy at the site of a stricture should be considered and biopsies sent for histology at the time of operation.

Which important factors should be considered in the surgical treatment of peri-anal Crohn's?

Peri-anal involvement occurs in approximately 90% of Crohn's patients at some point during the course of the disease. Fistulae and peri-anal sepsis are often complex and recurrent. Simple abscesses should be drained as close to the anal verge as possible to reduce the potential for fistula formation. The patient's pre-existing faecal and flatus continence should be considered as disease flare-ups may worsen diarrhoea in patients with a disrupted sphincter mechanism. Setons, open drainage, fistula plugs and mucosal advancement flaps are all valid options in the treatment of Crohn's fistulae; however, faecal diversion may be necessary to improve the rate of resolution.

The appendix

What is the surface marking of the appendix?

McBurney's point: one-third of the way along a line joining the right anterior superior iliac spine to the umbilicus.

What is a Meckel's diverticulum, in what proportion of the population does it occur, and where is it commonly found?

This is a blind-ending tubular structure formed from a remnant of the vitello-intestinal duct. It may be adherent to the umbilicus or connected to the umbilicus by a fibrous remnant of the duct.

It is present in approximately 2% of the population, is approximately 5 cm (2 inches) long and is usually found 60 cm (2 ft) from the caecum.

Which proportion of appendixes lie in the retrocaecal position at operation?

Approximately 75% are retrocaecal, 20% are pelvic and 5% are retroileal. It is also notable that approximately 90% of normal appendixes are found in the retroileal position.

What is the blood supply to the appendix?

The appendicular artery – a branch of the ileocolic artery. It runs behind the terminal ileum and within the mesoappendix.

What is the 'bloodless fold of Treves'?

This is the small fold of peritoneum joining the terminal ileum to the base of the mesoappendix.

What are the differential diagnoses for an acute appendicitis?

Gastrointestinal	Terminal ileitis, mesenteric adenitis (children), inflamed Meckel's diverticulum, carcinoid tumour, diverticulitis, acute cholecystitis.
Gynaecological	Ovarian cyst torsion or rupture, ectopic pregnancy, pelvic inflammatory disease.
Urological	Ureteric colic, pyelonephritis, testicular torsion.
Other	Diabetic ketoacidosis, shingles, acute porphyria.

Which are the key aspects present in the history and examination findings of a patient with acute appendicitis?

Pain –– This often begins as central, localizing to the right iliac fossa. It is colicky in nature initially but becoming constant and worse on movement as localized peritonitis ensues.

Pyrexia –– This is usually low grade but may be higher and accompanied by signs of generalized sepsis if late stage or perforation present.

Anorexia –– Patients may report anorexia with occasional episodes of vomiting.

Examination findings –– Pain localized to RIF with local rebound and guarding. Psoas irritation and a positive Rovsing's sign (pain in RIF on palpation in LIF) may also be present.

Which laboratory and radiological tests may be important in the diagnosis?

Laboratory –– Raised inflammatory markers are usually present; however, very high WCC or CRP should raise suspicion of other pathology or perforation or late stage disease.

Ultrasonography (USS) or CT scanning –– Ultrasonography is usually performed on women of childbearing age where the diagnosis of acute appendicitis is one of several differentials. CT scanning is usually not performed unless there is suspicion of a mass in the right iliac fossa or the patient is of older age with a history that leaves a wide differential for alternative pathology.

Which potential complications should be discussed when obtaining a patient's consent for laparoscopic appendectomy?

Complications relating to laparoscopy –– Bowel, bladder, vascular injury, conversion to an open procedure and even laparotomy. Shoulder tip pain following pneumoperitoneum may also be mentioned prior to the procedure.

Related to procedure –– Potential to require small bowel or large bowel resection, postoperative ileus, late adhesions leading to small bowel obstruction.

General complications –– Bleeding, infection (wound, chest, urine, etc.).

Describe the approaches to an open appendectomy

Lanz incision –– This is an oblique incision just below McBurney's point and along Langher's lines.

Gridiron incision –– This is a muscle splitting transverse incision over McBurney's point.

Briefly describe the procedure of open appendectomy

- Either a Lanz or a gridiron incision is made.
- The layers of the abdominal wall are then divided either with sharp dissection with a scalpel or by diathermy. The layers seen sequentially are

skin, subcutaneous fat, Scarpa's fascia, external oblique aponeurosis, internal oblique, transversus abdominis, transversalis fascia and peritoneum. Muscle layers should be split in the direction of their fibres.

- The peritoneum should be carefully lifted and entered cautiously so as not to cause inadvertent bowel injury.
- Once the peritoneum is entered, a microbiology swab or peritoneal fluid culture should be taken.
- The caecum is carefully delivered through the incision (adhesions may need to be divided) and the appendix localized by tracing the taeniae from the caecum to their termination at the appendix.
- A window is created between the mesoappendix and the appendix and the mesoappendix is clamped and ligated.
- The appendicular base is crushed, transfixed and divided.
- The appendix is removed and sent for histology.
- The stump may then be buried.
- Intraperitoneal lavage may then be performed prior to closing the incision closed in layers. A drain may be left *in situ* in the presence of pus.

Colorectal malignancies

What is the incidence of colorectal cancer in the UK?

The overall crude incidence rate is 63.3 per 100 000 population (Cancer Research UK, 2007 data).

What are the three commonest sites in which colonic malignancies arise?

The commonest site is the rectum at approximately 29%. This is followed by the sigmoid at 18% and the caecum at 13%.

Which aetiological factors are associated with colonic neoplasia?

Genetic	Polyposis syndromes such as Familial Adenomatous Polyposis (FAP), Hereditary Non-Polyposis Colorectal Cancer (HNPCC or Lynch Syndrome), Gardner syndrome.
Environmental	Smoking, diet (high in red meat and low in fibre), high alcohol intake, obesity.
Inflammatory bowel disease	(UC > Crohn's)

Infectious	There is some evidence to suggest that a link between chronic inflammation secondary to the presence of gut microflora may predispose to sporadic colorectal cancer. These bacteria include *Streptococcus bovis* and *Enterococcus faecalis*.

What is the adenoma-carcinoma sequence?

This describes the sequential progression from normal to dysplastic epithelial changes to malignant neoplasms as a result of multiple, sequential mutations in oncogenes, tumour suppressor and DNA mismatch repair genes. Key genes involved in the sequence include APC (adenomatous polyposis coli), K-ras and p53.

APC (tumour suppressor gene) –– The progression from normal to dysplastic epithelium is thought to occur as a result of mutation in the APC gene. APC gene mutations are seen in small adenomatous lesions, providing evidence for its role early in the adenoma-carcinoma sequence.

K-ras (oncogene) –– The oncogene K-ras is involved in the regulatory pathways of normal cell differentiation and proliferation. Mutations in the K-ras oncogene result in continuated activation of the Ras membrane protein. They appear to occur early in the development of small to large adenomas.

p53 –– p53 prevents the propagation of damaged DNA through several mechanisms, including blocking the proliferation of damaged DNA, stimulating DNA repair and, where this is not possible, stimulating apoptosis.

How is Lynch syndrome inherited and what is the genetic anomaly?

Autosomal dominant. The syndrome occurs due to a mutation in DNA mismatch repair genes (MSH2, MLH1, MSH6, PMS2), which results in microsatellite instability. Approximately 1–5% of all colorectal cancers are thought to occur as a result of mismatch repair-gene defects.

Which other cancers have been associated with Lynch syndrome?

Other cancers include: endometrial, ovarian, small bowel, stomach, renal tract, brain and skin. Patients with Lynch syndrome often also develop multiple tumours.

What are the revised Amsterdam criteria?

The Amsterdam criteria identify families who should be referred for genetic counselling and testing. All first-degree relatives in families with confirmed Lynch syndrome should be referred for colonoscopic surveillance. The four criteria are as follows:

1. At least three relatives have been diagnosed with colorectal or other HNPCC-associated cancer, one being a first-degree relative of the other two.

2. Two successive generations are affected.

3. One or more colonic cancers are diagnosed at age <50 years.

4. FAP has been excluded.

How is FAP inherited? What is the genetic anomaly?

FAP is an autosomal dominant condition associated with a mutation in the APC tumour-suppressor gene (Ch 5q21). MYH-polyposis may also be considered as a subset of FAP in some texts, and is caused by a mutation in the MUTYH gene (DNA repair). This is associated with an autosomal recessive pattern of inheritance.

What are the key features of FAP?

Multiple adenomas −− Develop in the second decade of life and are numerous (hundreds to thousands). Adenomas most commonly occur in the colon and rectum.

Extracolonic manifestations −− Osteomas, congenital hypertrophy of the retinal pigment epithelium (CHRPE), cutaneous lesions (lipomas, sebaceous cysts, epidermal cysts), dental abnormalities (unerupted, absent or supernumary teeth, odontomas or dental cysts).

Extracolonic malignancies −− Desmoid tumours, thyroid, primary hepatic, biliary and CNS tumours.

What is the risk of developing colorectal cancer in FAP patients left untreated?

The risk of developing malignancy is almost 100%. These tumours usually develop by age 40 years.

How might colonic malignancies present clinically?

Presentation is dependent on the site of the tumour. The key features associated with colonic malignancy include:

General −− Weight loss, cachexia, anorexia and malaise.

Specific −− Change in bowel habit, tenesmus, bleeding or mucous per rectum (proximal tumours may present with more occult bleeding (FOB+, Fe deficiency), whereas more distal malignancies often result in fresh or altered bleeding PR). Blood is often mixed with the stool.

Clinical examination −− Anaemia, jaundice, palpable abdominal mass, hepatomegaly (due to metastases) or ano-rectal mass per rectum.

Emergency –– Late-stage tumours may present with obstruction (large bowel obstruction more common in left-sided or rectal cancers), proximal right-sided malignancies may present with small bowel obstruction, perforation or acute peritonitis.

Metastatic disease –– Liver (pain, jaundice, palpable mass, altered LFTs), bone pain, pleural effusions or ascites.

Which investigations are available in the diagnosis of colonic malignancies?

Blood tests –– Iron deficiency anaemia, derangement of LFTs in hepatic metastases.

Tumour markers –– CEA and CA19–9. Used in determining prognosis and surveillance following resection.

Rigid sigmoidoscopy –– Used in a clinic setting for rapid assessment of the rectum. Able to assess up to 20cm. Biopsy samples may be obtained.

Flexible sigmoidoscopy –– Allows visualization of the colonic mucosa up to 60 cm (splenic flexure), therefore does not rule out proximal colonic malignancies. In the setting of colorectal cancer, flexible sigmoidoscopy is often used for surveillance of the anastomotic site following resection.

Colonoscopy –– The 'gold standard'. Enables full surveillance of the colon with biopsy of suspicious lesions and histopathological diagnosis. May be limited by the patient's co-morbidities and tolerance of bowel preparation regimens.

CT pneumocolon –– CT pneumocolon is beneficial in patients unable to tolerate colonoscopy or where colonoscopy has been incomplete. It also enables visualization of other sites of potential metastatic spread. Disadvantages include the inability to distinguish between hyperplastic and adenomatous polyps or to give histological diagnosis and a lower sensitivity than colonoscopy that may not reliably diagnose polyps <5mm in size.

Double contrast barium enema (DCBE) –– Once the 'gold-standard', DCBE has been largely superseded by CT colonography as CT is both more accurate, enables visualization of sites of distant metastases and involves lower radiation doses than DCBE.

2-[18F]fluoro-2-deoxy-d-glucose (2-FDG) PET-CT –– Uses the principle of increased glucose utilization by cancer cells to highlight malignant 'hot-spots'. PET alone is limited by lack of anatomical definition and the potential for increased uptake by non-malignant processes, such as infection. The combination of PET with CT therefore adds anatomical definition and information about other potential disease processes. This technique is particularly useful in staging and monitoring the response to treatment.

Briefly describe the key points of the national bowel cancer screening programme in the UK.

The national bowel cancer screening programme in the UK was first introduced in 2006 and became nationwide in 2010. All patients aged 60–69 are sent invitations to screening. Those accepting are sent a faecal occult blood (FOB) kit. Patients aged ≥70 may request FOB testing up to every two years. The FOB kit involves two samples taken from three separate bowel motions. It is completed by the patient at home and returned by post to the screening laboratory. Where the results are unclear or the test is performed incorrectly, the patient is sent a repeat kit. For each abnormal FOB test result, the patient is called to visit a specialist nurse at the GP surgery. At this point, a decision is made to refer the patient for colonoscopy if this appropriate, based on the history, examination and the patient's co-morbidities. Those patients with normal colonoscopy findings are then offered a further FOB test in two years if <70. Where colonoscopy findings indicate adenoma but no evidence of malignancy, the following recommendations have been made:

Low risk   one or two adenomas <1cm: repeat FOB testing in two years,

Intermediate risk   three or four adenomas <1cm or one adenoma ≥1cm: three-yearly colonoscopy surveillance until two negative examinations,

High risk   five or more adenomas <1cm or three or more adenomas of which at least one is ≥1cm: colonoscopy in twelve months followed by three-yearly colonoscopies until two negative examinations.

What is the Dukes staging system for colonic cancer?

Originally described by Cuthbert E. Dukes at St Mark's Hospital in 1932, the Dukes classification was originally developed for rectal cancer. It is now used to describe both colonic and rectal cancer and has been modified as follows:

Dukes A   Confined to the colon or rectal wall (overall five-year survival 92%),

Dukes B   Extends through the rectal wall into the peri-colonic or rectal tissue (five-year survival 77%),

Dukes C   Involves regional lymph nodes (five-year survival 47%),

Dukes D   Distant metastases (five-year survival 6%).

Note: Dukes D was not described in the original classification but was added later.

Describe the TNM staging of colorectal cancer

T0   No evidence of primary,

Tis   Carcinoma *in situ*,

T1   Invasion into the submucosa,

T2   Invasion into the muscularis propria,

T3   Invasion through the muscularis propria into the subserosa,

T4   Invasion into surrounding extracolonic structures or perforates the visceral peritoneum,

N0   No nodal involvement,

N1   1–3 peri-colic nodes involved,

N2 $\geq$4 peri-colic nodes involved,

N3   Distant nodal metastases,

M0   No distant metastases,

M1   Distant metastases.

Describe the key points in the non-surgical management of colonic cancer

Chemotherapy –– Adjuvant therapy is used in stage III and high-risk (evidence of vascular invasion or poorly differentiated tumours) stage II disease. Combination therapy with FOLFOX (5-Fluorouracil, folinic acid and oxaliplatin) improves disease-free survival at both three and five years and reduces the rates of disease recurrence (MOSAIC II trial).

Biological agents –– These are monoclonal antibodies (mAB), which may be used either as single agents or in combination with chemotherapeutic regimens, usually in patients with metastatic disease. Examples include Bevacizumab (a mAB against vascular endothelial growth factor (VEGF)) and Cetuximab or Panituximab (mABs against epithelial growth factor receptor (EGFR)).

Radiotherapy –– The role of radiotherapy is largely limited to resectable rectal cancer and the treatment of local metastatic disease (namely brain and bone metastases). In addition, it is recommended that primary chemo-radiotherapy be offered to patients with unresectable but non-metastatic rectal carcinoma, where they are medically fit. The tumour may then be re-staged and potentially curative resection considered if appropriate.

What is the role of neo-adjuvant therapy in the treatment of rectal cancer?

Pre-operative neo-adjuvant radiotherapy aims to reduce the risk of recurrence (short-course radiotherapy) or to shrink the tumour prior to resection (conventional fractionation). It is recommended that short-course radiotherapy be considered in all patients with resectable rectal cancer. Surgery should then be performed within one week of its completion. Where the aim is to downstage the tumour, radiotherapy is typically given over five weeks in conjunction with chemotherapy. Surgery is then performed six to eight weeks after its completion (ACPGBI guidelines). The disadvantages of neo-adjuvant therapy include peri-operative complications secondary to radiation injury (e.g., anastomotic breakdown) and a delay in performing a definitive surgical procedure. It is also notable that neo-adjuvant radiotherapy may only confer a marginal survival benefit. Postoperative adjuvant radiotherapy may be used as a salvage approach where there are positive resection margins and the patient has not received pre operative radiotherapy.

Which surgical strategies are available?

The choice of colonic resection depends on the site of the tumour. Ultimately, surgical resection provides the only curative treatment in colonic neoplasia. In suitable patients with Dukes D or Stage IV disease, metastatectomy in combination with resection of the primary tumour and adjuvant chemotherapy may be potentially curative. Successful resection is dependent on adequate resection margins (attaining an R0 resection) and sampling of associated lymphatics (a minimum of 12 associated LN). The anastomosis should be tension-free with a good vascular supply. Both open and laparoscopic treatment strategies are available and have comparative postoperative disease free survival and recurrence rates.

Site of tumour	Procedure	Arteries divided
Caecum and ascending colon	Right hemicolectomy	Ileocolic artery; right colic artery; right branch of middle colic arteries
Proximal to mid transverse colon	Extended right hemicolectomy	Ileocolic artery; right colic artery; middle colic artery (before bifurcation)
Splenic flexure to descending colon	Left hemicolectomy	Left branch of the middle colic artery; inferior mesenteric artery (IMA)
Sigmoid colon	Sigmoid colectomy	The IMA is ligated at its trunk and the splenic flexure is mobilized

Site of tumour	Procedure	Arteries divided
Rectum	Anterior resection (level depends on site of rectal tumour: low anterior resection is below the level of the peritoneal reflection)	IMA The ascending left colic branch of the IMA may be spared; however, the splenic flexure often needs to be mobilized to allow sufficient length to perform a tension free anastomosis

What are the complications of surgical resection of colonic tumours?

Immediate –– Bleeding, injury to surrounding structures (ureters, bladder, gonadal vessels, hypogastric nerve plexus, small bowel).

Early –– Infection, urinary retention (bladder denervation or direct injury), anastomotic leak, ileus.

Late –– Erectile dysfunction, anastomotic stricture, recurrence.

Chapter

15

The rectum and anus

Fissure *in ano*

Define fissure *in ano*

Fissure *in ano* is a longitudinal tear in the epithelial skin and anal mucosa, most commonly in the posterior (6 o'clock) position. Fissures may occur in the 12 o'clock position in approximately 10% of cases and are more common in women following childbirth.

What is the underlying pathophysiology of this condition?

It is thought that the initial insult may involve traumatic injury, e.g., from the passage of hard stool. However, in the majority of cases this heals without leading to development of a chronic anal fissure. It is likely that, in those patients developing anal fissure, there is an underlying abnormality of the internal anal sphincter leading to hypertonicity. This spasm exacerbates the relative ischaemia of the anodermal mucosa posteriorly and as a result can lead to the development of a fissure.

List the presenting features of fissure *in ano*

1. Bright red rectal bleeding, often on the toilet paper after wiping,
2. Painful defecation ('passing glass') and constipation,
3. Pruritis ani (rarely).

Which features may be seen on examination?

Anal sphincter spasm and pain may prevent full examination of the fissure. A sentinel skin tag may also be present, indicating a chronic fissure. Where the fissure may be visualized, the white fibres of the internal anal sphincter may be seen at the base of the fissure.

Which medical treatments are available for treatment of anal fissure?

Laxatives and bulking agents, e.g., fibrogel –– These will reduce constipation and soften stool.

GTN ointment, 0.2% BD –– This is used for a minimum trial of four weeks to relax the internal sphincter spasm, improve healing and reduce pain. Side effects, such as dizziness and headache may limit use.

Diltiazem, 2% BD –– This has been shown to be successful at reducing spasm and precipitating healing. Success rates have been shown to be as high as 75% after three months of therapy.

What surgical options are available?

Botulinum toxin (Botox) –– This is injected into the internal sphincter usually in the 3 o'clock and 9 o'clock positions under general anaesthesia, Botox blocks the sympathetic neuronal output of the internal anal sphincter, reducing excitatory tone. The effects of Botox are largely temporary; however, it has been shown to improve healing rates significantly when compared with controls. Documented side effects include flatus and faecal incontinence (often temporary but may be permanent), peri-anal haematoma and infection.

Lateral sphincterotomy –– Performed by either an open or a closed technique, this procedure involves partial division of the internal anal sphincter away from the fissure (usually in the 3 o'clock position). Risks include flatus and faecal incontinence (faecal incontinence was worse in older techniques where the incision was extended up to the dentate line). Success rates are, however, good and reported up to 95%.

Advancement flap –– This option may be suitable in patients with normal or hypotonic anal sphincters, where sphincterotomy may not be of benefit.

It is worth noting that both the anal stretch procedure and posterior sphincterotomy are no longer used, as both techniques give rise to a high risk of flatus and faecal incontinence.

Haemorrhoids

What are haemorrhoids and in which positions are they found?

Haemorrhoids represent engorgement of the fibrovascular cushions found within the anal canal. These areas within the submucosa have a rich arterio-venous supply, are supported by connective tissue and are consistently found in the 3, 7 and 11 o'clock positions. In the non-pathological situation, they act to form a watertight seal in the anal canal.

How are haemorrhoids classified?

Goligher classification system

Grade 1 Present with bleeding but no prolapse,

Grade 2 Prolapse and bleeding occurs but these spontaneously reduce,

Grade 3 Do not spontaneously reduce but may be reduced manually,

Grade 4 Continuously prolapsed and cannot be manually reduced.

Which non-surgical options are available in the management of haemorrhoids?

Dietary advice -- An increase in dietary fibre may increase stool bulk and improve constipation, which may have a role in the underlying aetiology of haemorrhoids.

Pharmacotherapy -- Stool softeners and laxatives.

Banding -- This may be carried out in either the operating theatre or the clinic setting in first-, second- or third-degree haemorrhoids. The haemorrhoid is identified and a suction device used to draw in the haemorrhoid at a level above the dentate line. A small rubber band is then fired around the base of the haemorrhoid. Research suggests that banding is likely to be more effective and require less re-intervention than sclerotherapy, although similar complications including bleeding and pain exist with banding.

Injection sclerotherapy (with 5% phenol in almond oil as sclerosant) -- Typically, this treatment is used in the outpatients setting for first- and second-degree symptomatic haemorrhoids. The sclerosant is injected above the dentate line into the base of the haemorrhoid to minimize discomfort. It should be noted that whilst this treatment improves bleeding from haemorrhoids it does not affect prolapse. Repeated treatments may be necessary, and a number of patients require other forms of treatment.

Photocoagulation -- This technique uses infrared coagulation to create ulceration at the base of the haemorrhoid and ultimately results in shrinkage of the haemorrhoidal mass. Its use is mainly limited to smaller non-prolapsing haemorrhoids and is dependent on the availability of equipment.

Which surgical options are available in the management of haemorrhoids?

Open haemorrhoidectomy -- This procedure involves excision of the haemorrhoids under general anaesthetic. The external portion of the haemorrhoid is excised with diathermy, and the remaining tissue dissected from the white fibres of the internal sphincter. Haemostasis of the vascular pedicle is achieved and the wounds are left to heal by secondary intention. Preservation of the skin bridges must be ensured to prevent stricturing.

Closed haemorrhoidectomy -- This involves the same procedure of excision as the open haemorrhoidectomy; however, the wounds are closed with absorbable suture following excision. There is some suggestion that closed haemorrhoidectomy may be associated with slightly reduced postoperative pain when compared with the open technique, however wound healing may be slower if dehiscence occurs. The overall outcomes are largely comparable between these techniques.

Stapled haemorrhoidopexy –– Suitable for both third- and fourth-degree haemorrhoids, this technique involves a circular stapled mucosectomy using a specialized device approximately 4 cm above the dentate line. The removal of this ring of tissue both disrupts the vascular supply to the haemorrhoids and shortens the degree of mucosal prolapse. Stapled haemorrhoidopexy may be associated with reduced postoperative pain when compared with the open techniques. Potential complications of rectal perforation, recto-vaginal fistula and pelvic sepsis are rare but have been reported.

Haemorrhoidal artery ligation operation (HALO) –– Usually performed under either sedation or general anaesthesia, this technique utilizes a miniature Doppler ultrasound device attached to a specially designed proctoscope to trans-anally localize the six main trunks of the haemorrhoidal artery. Once each trunk has been visualized, a suture is inserted through the device and used to ligate each vessel precisely within the rectal wall. The HALO technique is relatively new (introduced in 1995) and not performed in all centres. However, results are encouraging, with good long-term control of both bleeding and prolapse, as well as a low rate of recurrence.

Which complications may be associated with surgical haemorrhoidectomy?

Early –– Pain, bleeding, acute urinary retention, constipation, infection.

Late –– Recurrence, anal stenosis, faecal incontinence.

Fistula *in ano*

What is the definition of a fistula?

A fistula is an abnormal connection between two epithelial lined surfaces.

What is Goodsall's rule?

With the patient lying in the lithotomy position, an imaginary transverse line is drawn across the anus from the 9 o'clock to 3 o'clock positions. If an external opening is visible anterior to this line, the tract is likely to pass directly to the anal canal. If, however, the external opening is visible posterior to this line, the tract is likely to curve in a horseshoe fashion and the internal opening is likely to be in the midline posteriorly.

What is the underlying pathophysiology of peri-anal fistulae?

It is thought that fistulae often result from previous cryptoglandular sepsis drained either spontaneously or surgically. The remaining cavity and tract, lined with granulation tissue, may then develop into an established fistula. The internal opening of the fistula (within the rectum) is formed from the original opening of the gland, and the external opening is formed from the drainage site on the skin.

How may peri-anal fistulae be classified?

Park's classification (Figure 15.1)

Intersphincteric	Commonest (70%). The tract passes through the internal sphincter and runs in the intersphincteric space before opening onto the perineal skin.
Transphincteric	Approximately 25%. The course passes through the internal sphincter and then runs low through the superficial external sphincter to enter the ischiorectal fossa before opening onto the perineal skin.
Suprasphincteric	Less common (approximately 5%). The tract runs high through the internal sphincter and in the intersphincteric space, through the puborectalis and into the ischiorectal fossa before opening onto the perineum.

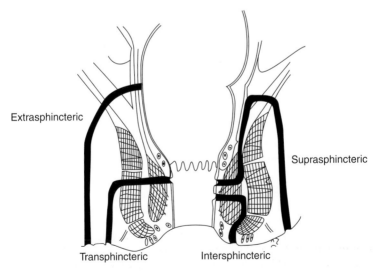

Figure 15.1 Park's classification of peri-anal fistulae.

Extrasphincteric   (<1%) These high fistulae are often associated with pelvic abscesses. The tract runs from the rectum, through the levator ani to the peri-anal skin and remains outside the sphincter complex.

It is worth noting that subcutaneous fistulae are not included in Park's classification as they are not usually of cryptoglandular origin.

Which surgical treatment options are available for the management of fistula *in ano*?

The initial management must focus on identifying the course of the fistula tract and any underlying disease process that may be responsible (e.g., Crohn's). In recurrent pelvic sepsis or patients with underlying IBD, imaging using pelvic MRI or transrectal USS is advised prior to intervention.

Surgical management can be broadly divided into the following techniques, although each should be preceded by formal examination of the tract or tracts under anaesthesia:

Lay open -- This may be used in submucosal, intersphincteric and low transphincteric fistulae. Care should be taken to probe the tract and confirm its relation to the sphincters. The tract is then opened completely, curetted and left to heal by secondary intention. Potential effects on continence should be discussed with the patient during consent.

Seton placement -- The purpose of a seton is to promote drainage, fibrosis and, in the case of a tight seton, slowly cut through the fistula whilst minimizing the effect on the sphincter mechanism. A cutting seton may be tightened at regular intervals over a 6–8 week period to stimulate healing. A loose seton serves the primary aim of providing drainage and reducing sepsis. A more definitive procedure is then usually required at a later date.

Fistula plug -- The fistula is defined and the tract probed and curetted. A conical plug of porcine intestinal submucosa is pulled into the tract until the internal opening is closed. This is then sutured in place. The external opening is left partially open to allow drainage to continue and the plug acts as a scaffold for new tissue growth.

Mucosal advancement flap -- This may be appropriate for patients with chronic high fistulae without evidence of significant sepsis. Complete excision of the primary and secondary fistula tracts is performed and a wide-based mucomuscular flap of rectum is raised and pulled down over the internal opening. The defect is closed and the flap sutured in place.

Of note, it may also be necessary to consider temporary defunctioning colostomy in the event of recurrent failure of treatment to allow healing to take place.

Pilonidal disease

What is a pilonidal sinus?

A pilonidal sinus is a blind-ended tract, most commonly in the natal cleft (although also observed in the finger pulp and interdigital spaces of barbers and sheep shearers), lined with stratified squamous epithelium and granulation tissue. A cyst cavity often develops at the base of the sinus, containing hair and epithelial debris. A chronic inflammatory reaction becomes established in the base of these pits with infiltration of neutrophil polymorphs, lymphocytes, plasma cells and macrophages.

What is the incidence of pilonidal disease and which age group does it most commonly affect?

The incidence of pilonidal disease in the general population is approximately 26 in 100 000. It most commonly affects young adults aged 16–25 years.

Briefly describe the pathogenesis of pilonidal sinus

A pilonidal sinus is thought to originate from distorted, enlarged hair follicles, creating keratin-filled pits within the natal cleft. Hair, skin debris and bacteria are then drawn into these pits, creating a foreign body reaction and generating micro-abscesses. Irritation from surrounding skin and hair causes recurrent infection, prevents healing and allows chronic infection to develop.

What are the common presenting features of pilonidal disease?

Whilst many pilonidal sinuses are asymptomatic, swelling and pain and purulent discharge in the natal cleft area are common presenting symptoms. Examination reveals the presence of one or more sacral pits, with or without associated abscess formation.

Which treatment options are available in the management of pilonidal sinus?

Conservative management –– Patients with asymptomatic disease without the presence of abscess or local infection may be reassured, with advice given to return should acute infection develop. To reduce the risk of recurrence, conservative management may also involve hair control by means of regular shaving of the natal cleft or laser depilation.

Surgical management –– The mainstay of surgical management in an acute pilonidal abscess is incision and drainage (with or without curettage) followed by packing and postoperative wound care. To prevent premature wound closure and recurrence of infection, the incision should be placed lateral to the midline, with or without the excision of a small 'button' of tissue (Bascom technique). These patients should then be followed up and a definitive procedure offered, to excise the pits and prevent recurrence of symptoms.

The principles of definitive surgical management involve excision of the sinus tract, adequate closure and healing and prevention of recurrence. Several techniques have been described, including:

1. Lay-open of sinus tract,
2. Excision with primary closure (off-midline),
3. Excision with marsupialization,
4. Excision and closure with cutaneous flap (Karydakis and Rhomboid or Limberg flaps).

Briefly describe the Limberg procedure.

A rhomboid incision is made over the sinus tract, extending down to the presacral fascia. The incision is then extended laterally to the gluteal fascia in the same dimensions as the area excised. Finally, a fascio-cutaneous flap is lifted from this lateral incision and transposed to perform a tension-free closure of the defect.

What is the Karydakis procedure?

A vertical elliptical incision is made to excise the sinus. By undermining the medial edge of the ellipse, a cutaneous flap is created, which is then advanced across the midline. Closure is performed in this lateral position, creating a vertical scar lateral to the midline. This technique aims to reduce the risk of recurrence and improve wound healing.

What are the complications of pilonidal sinus excision?

Early	Wound dehiscence, infection,
Immediate	Bleeding,
Late	Recurrence, scarring.

Anal malignancies

What is the incidence of anal cancer?

The overall age-adjusted incidence rate is 1.5 per 100 000 in the USA. The incidence is higher in women than in men.

Which aetiological factors are associated with an increased risk of anal cancer?

Human papilloma virus infection	particularly subtype HPV-16.
Immunosuppression	Following solid organ transplantation, immunosuppression increases the risk of squamous cell carcinoma.
Smoking.	

| Sexual practice and HIV | Epidemiological data suggest a link between anal intercourse and anal cancer. As yet, the link between HIV and anal cancer is unproven and, rather than being causal, may reflect the higher rates of HPV infection and immunosuppression in the HIV$^+$ population. It is also notable that the prevalence of anal cancer in HIV$^+$ patients has not shown a decrease since the advent of HAART. |

Which histological subtypes are found in anal cancer?

Squamous cell carcinoma (70%)	Originates from the squamous mucosa of the lower anal canal or more rarely the anal transition zone. Squamous cell carcinoma may be divided into large-cell keratinizing, large cell non-keratinizing and basaloid subtypes.
Adenocarcinoma (10%)	Usually has the same phenotype as rectal carcinoma and arises from the upper anal canal or the anal transition zone. Adenocarcinoma may also arise from the anal ducts, within anorectal fistulae or in the form of intraepithelial adenocarcinoma (anal Paget's disease).
Neuroendocrine	
Malignant melanoma (4%)	
Other	Including mesenchymal tumours and lymphomas.

How might anal cancer present clinically?

Rectal bleeding and pain are the most common presenting features. Bleeding is usually bright red and may be misdiagnosed as being due to haemorrhoidal disease. Rectal pain and fullness may also be present.

What is the role of endoanal ultrasound (EAUS) and MRI scanning in the diagnosis and staging of anal cancer?

Endoanal ultrasound (EAUS) –– This is used in the assessment of the extent of local disease, in particular T1 and T2 stage lesions. It is usually well tolerated, cheap and safe. Its use may be limited in stenotic tumours. It is, however, less useful in looking at mesorectal lymph node involvement.

MRI –– This is used to assess the extent of local disease spread and invasion of surrounding sphincter complex and urethral or vaginal involvement. It also allows assessment of peri-rectal nodal involvement.

Briefly describe the key principles involved in the non-surgical management of anal cancer

Chemoradiotherapy is the mainstay of oncological management in anal carcinoma. Chemotherapy is most commonly by combination treatment with 5-FU and mitomycin. Combination chemo- and radiotherapy is more effective than radiotherapy alone.

Which regional lymph nodes may be the site of metastatic spread in anal cancer?

Above the dentate line, lymphatic drainage of the anal canal is to the paravertebral and peri-rectal nodes and these may be the site of lymphatic spread in anal cancer. This differs from tumours below the dentate line where the inguinal, femoral and internal iliac nodes are affected.

What are the indications for abdomino-perineal resection (APER)?

1. Rectal tumours with evidence of involvement of the sphincter complex or where the tumour is too low to achieve sufficient margins of clearance without APER.
2. Residual or recurrent anal tumour following chemoradiotherapy.

Briefly describe the principles of open APER

The patient is commonly positioned in the Lloyd–Davies position and the abdomen initially approached via a lower midline laparotomy incision. The procedure can be divided into the abdominal phase and the perineal phase.

Abdominal phase The first stage of the procedure involves mobilization of the left colon and sigmoid. The inferior mesenteric artery and vein are identified and divided. Care is taken to visualize the left ureter and gonadal vessels to avoid inadvertent injury. The dissection is then continued to mobilize the rectum in the TME plane to the level of the levator ani complex. It is important to avoid injury to the hypogastric plexus of nerves and ureters at this stage.

Perineal phase A purse string suture is placed around the anus and pulled tight to close the anus. An elliptical incision is made approximately 3 cm from the anus and the anococcygeal ligament is divided posteriorly. The incision is then continued deep through the levator sling to reach the level of the abdominal dissection, the middle and inferior rectal vessels are identified and ligated.

The colon may then be divided (usually through the abdominal incision) and the anus and rectum are removed through the perineal wound. An end colostomy is formed to terminalize the colon. The left and right pelvic diaphragms are sutured to close the perineal defect and the perineal skin is closed with an absorbable subcuticular suture. Perineal and pelvic drains are placed, and mass closure of the abdominal wound is performed.

Note The perineal phase of this procedure is now increasingly performed in the prone position. This enables a more extensive perineal dissection with excision of a wider, 'cylindrical' area of ischiorectal fat and levator muscle, in an attempt to reduce the rates of local recurrence. This may however result in difficulty with adequate closure and may necessitate creation of a gluteal or rectus abdominis flap.

What are the complications of APER?

Immediate –– Bleeding (often from presacral veins), ureteric injury, rectal perforation, hypogastric nerve injury.

Early –– Perineal wound dehiscence, bladder dysfunction (may be incomplete emptying, incontinence, urgency or loss of sensation of bladder filling and is associated with damage to hypogastric plexus of nerves), erectile dysfunction, retrograde ejaculation, infection, stoma related complications (ischaemia or necrosis, prolapse or retraction).

Late –– Perineal hernia, recurrence (increased recurrence rates may be associated with intra-operative rectal perforation), complications related to the stoma (prolapse, retraction, hernia).

Chapter 16

The kidneys and genitourinary system

Renal calculi

What is the commonest composition of renal calculi?

Calcium oxalate with calcium phosphate.

Which other types of renal stones may form?

Among the rarer type of renal stone, the most frequently identified include: magnesium ammonium phosphate (struvite), cystine and uric acid stones.

Briefly describe the key points in the pathophysiology of development of renal calculi

Supersaturation –– The development of renal calculi is most commonly due to supersaturation of the urine, with a high ratio of calcium oxalate to calcium phosphate allowing crystals to nucleate and grow and for stones to form. Calcium phosphate supersaturation increases with increase in urinary pH.

Anatomical abnormalities –– (Such as pelvi-ureteric junction obstruction, horseshoe kidney and polycystic kidney disease.) These increase urinary stasis and promote stone formation.

Metabolic factors –– Hypercalciuria (familial, dietary or idiopathic); hyperparathyroidism, increased oxalate absorption.

Hypocitraturia –– (For example, due to renal tubular acidosis, carbonic anhydrase inhibitors.) This reduces the chelation effect of citrate on calcium in the urine.

Hyperuricosuria –– (For example, high dietary purine intake.) Increased calcium stone formation due to reduced calcium oxalate solubility.

What is the prevalence of renal calculi?

Approximately 11% men and 5–6% women by the age of 70 develop renal calculi (USA).

What are the commonest sites of obstruction due to renal stones?

The three commonest sites of obstruction are the pelvi-ureteric junction, the pelvic brim and the vesico-ureteric junction. These represent the narrow areas of the urinary tract.

What are the common features in the presentation of renal stone disease?

- Pain: clinical features may vary with the site of obstruction, although severe, colicky loin-groin pain that is worse on remaining still is the classically described presentation. Pelvi-ureteric stones may present with deep flank pain without radiation to the groin, whereas ureteric stones may present with a severe colicky pain radiating to the groin and ipsilateral testicle or the vulva. Vesico-ureteric stones may cause urinary frequency and urgency.
- Nausea and vomiting.
- Microscopic haematuria.

Which key investigations are important in the diagnosis of renal stone disease?

Blood tests –– Renal function – knowledge of renal impairment is important both to assess organ dysfunction and prior to giving contrast agents for imaging. Raised inflammatory markers, pyrexia and pyuria may indicate urinary tract infection or more seriously pyelonephrosis. Serum calcium and urate should be measured and PTH checked in the presence of hypercalcaemia.

Plain kidney–ureter–bladder (KUB) radiography and intravenous uretogram (IVU) –– Plain KUB alone has a low sensitivity and specificity for diagnosis of renal stones. An intravenous uretogram defines the anatomy of the collecting system, ureters and bladder and gives information on renal tract dilatation, as well as the position of obstruction. The disadvantages include the need for IV contrast with potential limitations in patients with renal dysfunction and the risk of contrast allergy.

CT-KUB –– This has a high sensitivity and specificity (sensitivity 95–100%) and removes the requirement for IV contrast. The other advantage is that information is provided about surrounding structures allowing screening of other potential pathology.

Ultrasound –– This allows visualization of the anatomical structure of the kidneys, assessment of stones and hydroureter, although it has a lower sensitivity and specificity than CT-KUB and IVU.

What percentage of renal calculi are radio-opaque?

85–90%.

What are the medical treatment options in the management of nephrolithiasis?

Uncomplicated nephrolithiasis, in the absence of infection, obstruction or renal dysfunction can usually be managed with analgesia (NSAIDs may be particularly beneficial in reducing ureteric spasm) and fluid replacement where dehydration is present.

What percentage of renal stones pass spontaneously?

This is dependent on the position of the stone within the renal tract and the size of the stone. When all positions are considered:

≤5 mm	68% pass spontaneously,
>5 mm but <10 mm	47% pass spontaneously,
≥10 mm	Unlikely to pass spontaneously, guidelines recommend surgical intervention.

What are the indications for surgical intervention?

The key indications for surgical intervention are:
1. Increasing or unremitting pain (despite analgesic therapy),
2. Obstruction in the presence of infection,
3. Risk of pyelonephritis or urosepsis,
4. Failure of stone progression,
5. Obstruction in a solitary kidney,
6. Bilateral obstruction.

Which surgical treatment strategies are available?

In patients presenting with obstruction and associated infection, urgent drainage is required by means of percutaneous nephrostomy or retrograde ureteric stent placement.

Extra-corporeal shock wave lithotripsy (ESWL) –– The patient is either sedated or under general anaesthesia during the procedure. The principle of ESWL is as follows: an external, high-frequency acoustic pulse is delivered using either an electromagnetic, electrohydraulic or piezoelectric device. A shock wave is produced by the release of high-energy over a small area. Once the stone has been located by either ultrasound or fluoroscopy, the delivery of focused shock waves produces a shear stress across the calculus, resulting in its fragmentation.

Ureteroscopic lithotripsy (URS) –– Both ureteroscopic lithotripsy and ESWL are accepted first-line treatments, although stone-free rates may be higher with the ureteroscopic approach. The rigid ureteroscope is passed via the urethra and bladder into the ureter, enabling direct visualization of the calculus. Laser lithotripsy may then be used to fragment the stone and the fragments removed either with a grasper or by using a retrieval basket. Following the procedure, a ureteral stent may be inserted. Whilst ureteral stenting is not required in all cases, complications, such as ureteral injury, stricture, renal dysfunction and significant residual stones, may necessitate stent placement.

Retrograde intrarenal surgery (RIRS) -- Under fluoroscopic guidance, a guidewire is placed transurethrally into the renal pelvis. The flexible ureteroscope is passed over the guidewire and systematic examination of the pelvi-calyceal system is carried out. Lithotripsy is then performed and stone fragments collected with a retrieval basket or grasper. As with URS, a stent may be placed at the end of the procedure.

Percutaneous nephrolithotomy -- Percutaneous stone retrieval may be particularly useful for large, renal pelvis stones (e.g., staghorn calculi) and some upper ureteric stones. In cases of upper ureteric stones where ESWL and ureteroscopy have failed, it may also be used as a second-line treatment. The principle of an antegrade approach is as follows: a needle is inserted through the posterolateral aspect of the flank into the desired calyx under ultrasound or fluoroscopic guidance. A guidewire is then passed through the needle and into the collecting system as far as the pelvic ureter. The tract is then widened with a series or dilators and a sheath placed to allow passage of the nephroscope directly into the kidney. Stone retrieval may then be performed directly with graspers or after use of lithotripsy techniques to fragment larger stones.

Open or laparoscopic uretolithotomy -- This is reserved for cases where ESWL, ureteroscopy or percutaneous stone retrieval have failed, or for complex stone burden.

Briefly list the complications associated with surgical intervention for urinary calculi

General
- Urinary sepsis,
- Bleeding.

Specific
- Stent pain, migration, breakage or obstruction,
- Extravasation of irrigation fluid into retroperitoneal space during percutaneous approaches,
- Ureteric injury and extravasation of irrigation fluid during uretroscopy,
- Damage to surrounding peritoneum, bowel, spleen, pleura or vascular structures during percutaneous or open approaches,
- Obstruction secondary to residual stone burden or remaining stone fragments.

Renal and urinary tract malignancies

What is the commonest type of renal malignancy?

Renal cell carcinoma (RCC) (90% of all renal malignancies).

What is the classical triad of presentation of renal cell carcinoma?

The classical triad consists of: loin pain, palpable loin mass and visible (macroscopic) haematuria. It occurs rarely and >50% of renal tumours are incidental findings during imaging for non-specific symptoms.

What is the significance of a varicocele in renal cancer?

Invasion of the left renal vein by tumour may lead to occlusion of the left testicular vein and 'back pressure' on the pampiniform plexus of veins resulting in a non-reducing varicocele. This typically does not occur on the right side, as the gonadal vein drains directly into the inferior vena cava.

What are the commonest sites of metastases?

- Lung (Commonest approx. 75%),
- Soft tissue (35%),
- Bone (20%),
- Liver (18%),
- Cutaneous (5–10%),
- CNS.

Which aetiological factors are associated with an increased risk of renal cell carcinoma?

1. *Genetic*: Von Hipple Lindau Syndrome (approx. 40% develop RCC); tuberous sclerosis; positive family history in first-degree relative,
2. *Lifestyle*: Smoking, obesity,
3. Acquired cystic disease of the kidney.

What are the commonest pathological subtypes of renal cell carcinoma?

Clear cell	Commonest (80–90%); usually arises in the proximal renal tubule.
Papillary	Second most common (10–15%); usually multifocal and often bilateral. Also arises from the proximal tubule.
Chromatophobe	(4–5%); arises from the cortical collecting duct.

What is the Bosniak classification system?

First proposed by Bosniak in 1986, this classification system is used to categorize renal cysts according to their appearance on ultrasound or CT:

Class I   Benign lesions that do not require surgical intervention.

Class II   A typically benign cyst. A few hairline septa and fine calcification may be present; however, the lesion is sharply marginated and non-enhancing.

Class IIf   These cysts contain more features suspicious of malignancy. More significant septation may be present with evidence of calcification. There are no enhancing soft-tissue elements.

Class III   These are complicated lesions displaying some features of malignancy. They appear as indeterminate cystic masses with an irregular, thickened wall and evidence of septation and calcification. Surgical exploration is usually required.

Class IV   These represent malignant lesions that require surgical resection.

Distinguishing between benign and malignant cysts by USS or CT alone is often difficult. A number of lesions classified into group II are ultimately found to be malignant and a number classified into group III may turn out to be benign.

Briefly describe the TNM staging system for renal carcinoma

T1   1a – $\leq$4 cm; 1b – >4 cm and $\leq$7 cm; limited to the kidney.

T2   >7 cm; limited to the kidney.

T3   3a – Peri-nephric fat or adrenal invasion; 3b – infradiaphragmatic renal vein or vena cava involvement. T3 lesions do not breach Gerota's fascia.

T4   Invasion extends beyond Gerota's fascia and involves the supra-diaphragmatic vena cava.

N1   One regional lymph node involved.

N2   More than one regional lymph node involved.

M0   No distant metastases.

M1   Distant metastases (typically bone, cerebral).

Briefly describe the management of renal cell carcinoma

Radical nephrectomy –– This may be performed either open or laparoscopically. The kidney is resected 'en bloc' with its associated peri-nephric fat, adrenal gland and Gerota's fascia. Lymph-node dissection may also be performed. In the presence of renal vein metastases, the renal artery is ligated early with minimal manipulation of the renal vein. Involvement of the IVC requires control of the vessel above and below the lesion, resection of the thrombus or lesion and subsequent repair of the IVC. The benefit of the laparoscopic approach is improved wound healing, lower risk of incisional hernia formation, earlier return to work and reduced postoperative pain. Disadvantages include potential spillage of malignant cells or spread along port site tracts and concern over the risk of positive resection margins.

Nephron-sparing surgery (partial nephrectomy) –– Typically used to treat T1a and 1b lesions, the aim of nephron sparing surgery is to preserve renal function while still obtaining adequate oncological clearance.

Radiofrequency ablation and cryotherapy –– A needle probe is inserted percutaneously into the tumour under fluoroscopic guidance. Either radiofrequency or cryothermic energy is then used to ablate the tumour cells. This technique may be effective in small localized renal masses or where the patient may be unsuitable for partial nephrectomy. It is potentially curative.

What is the treatment of metastatic renal cell carcinoma?
Surgical –– Radical nephrectomy.

Radiotherapy –– Renal cell carcinoma is largely radioresistant. Therefore, radiotherapy is reserved for palliation and control of metastatic disease not responding to systemic treatment (largely cerebral and bony metastases).

Systemic treatments
- *Chemotherapy*: RCC shows poor response rates ($<15\%$) to standard chemotherapeutic agents. An example regimen includes gemcitabine and 5-Fluorouracil.
- *Immunotherapy*: Interleukin-2 (IL-2) (high dose), Interferon alpha (IFN-α).
- mTOR kinase inhibitors (e.g., temsirolimus).

Renal artery embolization –– Control of haematuria and flank pain.

Urinary tract and bladder malignancies
What are the commonest histological subtypes of bladder cancer in the developed world?
Bladder tumours are almost all of urothelial origin. The commonest (90%) is transitional cell carcinoma (TCC), followed by squamous cell carcinoma (5%) and adenocarcinoma (1–2%).

What other aetiological factors may be associated with urothelial tumours?

Occupational	Aromatic (aryl) amines in dyes, solvents and textiles.
Smoking	Is associated with 50–65% of urothelial tumours in men and 20–30% in women.

Urinary stone disease	Chronic irritation secondary to stone disease may predispose to squamous cell carcinoma.
Drugs	Chemotherapeutic, agents such as cyclophosphamide.
Iatrogenic	Long-term indwelling urinary catheters may cause chronic irritation and predispose to squamous cell carcinoma.
Genetic	Urothelial tumours are generally non-hereditary. An exception to this is Lynch syndrome II (colonic and urothelial malignancies).
Environmental	Squamous cell carcinoma may be secondary to chronic inflammation from *Schistosoma haematobium* infection.

Which clinical features may be associated with bladder cancer?

- *Painless frank haematuria*: Should be considered a warning sign of bladder malignancy until proven otherwise,
- Dysuria,
- Urgency,
- Frequency,
- *Symptoms of metastatic spread*: Bone pain, flank pain (ureteric obstruction), pelvic pain (local invasion).

What is the gold-standard diagnostic test in suspected bladder malignancy?

Cystoscopy. This identifies gross urothelial abnormalities and visualization of papillary and flat lesions. It is notable that the macroscopic appearance of carcinoma *in situ* may be similar to chronic inflammation.

Which urinary tests have been used as biomarkers in the diagnosis and surveillance of bladder cancer?

1. Urinary cytology (useful in high-grade malignancy and carcinoma *in situ*),
2. Nuclear matrix protein (NMP-22),
3. Bladder tumour antigen (BTA).

Briefly describe the procedure of transurethral resection of bladder tumours (TURBT)

TURBT is both diagnostic and therapeutic. It is usually performed under general anaesthesia. A cystoscope is passed transurethrally into the bladder and a systematic cystoscopy is performed. Directed biopsies should be taken of any area of suspicious or inflamed urothelium to exclude carcinoma *in situ*. Visible lesions are resected by electrocautery and sent for histology. Muscle EUA should be performed to evaluate the presence of a palpable mass (mobile or fixed) indicating muscle invasive disease. Following TURBT a single shot of intravesical chemotherapy may be given to reduce recurrence thought to occur as a result of tumour cell dispersal following TURBT. This should be avoided in cases complicated by perforation of significant ongoing bleeding requiring irrigation.

Which key features of the tumour should be noted following TURBT?

1. *Location*: base, dome, trigone or lateral wall,
2. *Type of tumour*: Papillary or solid,
3. Size,
4. Number of tumours,
5. Residual mass on EUA.

What are the complications of TURBT?

Early –– Haemorrhage requiring continuous irrigation, perforation (extraperitoneal perforation may be managed conservatively, whilst intraperitoneal perforation may require laparotomy, open exploration and repair), TUR syndrome, urosepsis.

Late –– Recurrence, urethral stricturing due to scarring.

Which agents are used in the management of non-muscle invasive urothelial tumours?

BCG (bacillus Calmette-Guérin)	Increases Th1 response (IL-2 and IFN-α),
Mitomycin C	Inhibits DNA synthesis,
Doxorubicin	Inhibits DNA synthesis by inhibiting topoisomerase,
Interferon and BCG combination therapy	Increases Th-1 response, antiproliferative and antiangiogenic.

Briefly outline the management of muscle invasive urothelial tumours

Surgical –– Radical cystectomy is the 'gold-standard' treatment for stage T2–T4a muscle-invasive bladder cancer. The urinary bladder is removed along with all visible tumour, the distal ureters and local lymph nodes. In the female, complete pelvic exenteration also involves removal of the adjacent vagina and uterus. Where possible, preservation of the urethra, rhabdosphincter, intra-pelvic autonomic and sensory nerves should be performed to preserve function and allow for neobladder creation. In the male, the prostate and seminal vesicles may also be preserved. Following radical cystectomy, the method of urinary diversion may be variable, although most commonly either an ileal orthotopic neobladder or an ileal conduit is performed.

Chemotherapy –– Neo-adjuvant cisplatin-containing combination chemotherapy should be offered to all patients with muscle-invasive bladder cancer unless contraindicated. Chemotherapy may also be used in the treatment of non-resectable primary tumours, although a durable complete response is rarely achieved. First-line agents include a regimen of gemcitabine and cisplatin; or combination therapy with methotrexate, vinblastine, adriamycin, and cisplatin (European Association of Urology, 2011 guidelines).

Radiotherapy –– Pre-operative radiotherapy has been shown to lead to downstaging in muscle-invasive bladder cancer. However, the current evidence does not show a significant survival benefit and therefore pre-operative radiotherapy is not recommended in the 2011 guidelines.

The prostate

How is the prostate anatomically divided?

The prostate is divided into three zones: a peripheral zone (surrounding the central zone postero-inferiorly), a central zone (surrounding the ejaculatory ducts) and a transitional zone (around the distal preprostatic urethra).

Which of these zones is commonly affected in benign prostatic hypertrophy (BPH)?

The transition zone.

Which zone is the site of origin of most prostatic cancers?

The peripheral zone.

What is the lifetime risk of developing prostate cancer in the UK?

Prostate cancer is the commonest malignancy in men in the UK carrying a lifetime risk of one in nine and with a crude incidence of 122 per 100 000 (Cancer Research UK data).

What is the commonest histological subtype of prostatic cancer?

Acinar type adenocarcinoma (90%).

What are the rarer histological subtypes?

These include small-cell neuroendocrine tumours, adenoid cystic and basal cell tumours and squamous cell carcinomas. Urothelial, germ cell and sarcomatous carcinomas may also occur.

What is PSA?

Prostate-specific antigen (PSA) is a serum protease produced by the prostatic cells and excreted in the ejaculate fluid to participate in the dissolution of the seminal fluid coagulum. In the absence of prostatic disease, only small amounts of PSA are present in the serum; however, in the presence of cancer, disruption of the prostatic architecture leads to significantly elevated serum levels. Other prostatic disease, such as inflammation, trauma and BPH, may also lead to elevated PSA levels, as can urinary retention and urinary tract infections.

What is the role of PSA in prostate cancer screening?

There is no established prostate cancer-screening programme, as several multicentre trials (the Prostate, Lung, Colorectal and Ovarian Cancer Screening Trial and the European Randomised Study of Screening for Prostate Cancer) have failed to show a significant survival benefit with PSA screening. Current recommendations therefore advise that men should discuss the benefit of prostate cancer screening around age 40, in particular high-risk patients with a positive family history. A baseline PSA may then be taken and a digital rectal examination performed. The interval before follow-up screening is also debated and may range from every two years to every seven years.

How might prostate cancer present clinically?

Prostatic cancer is often picked up incidentally on PSA screening in the absence of overt clinical symptoms, or during investigation for lower urinary tract symptoms. However, clinical features of prostatic cancer may include urinary retention, back pain, leg pain, haematuria and reduced urinary stream.

What is the Gleason scoring system?

The Gleason score was originally proposed in 1966 and is a histological scoring system. It has been subject to several updates since then, most recently in 2005. Two Gleason grades are given, one to the most common tumour pattern within the sample and one to the second most common pattern. The sum of these two grades is the Gleason score. The grade assigned to each pattern ranges from 1–5:

Type 1   The architecture of the tumour tissue is close to that of the normal prostate. Small, closely packed and well-defined glands are visible.

Type 2   The glandular appearance is well defined but the glands themselves are larger and interspersed with a larger area of stromal tissue.

Type 3   Whilst discrete glands exist, there is marked irregularity in their size and shape. Tiny glands may have begun to invade the stroma.

Type 4   There is 'ragged infiltration' with almost complete loss of normal glandular architecture. Glands have become fused together with poorly formed glandular lumina and significant cellular invasion into surrounding tissue.

Type 5   There is complete loss of glandular architecture with extensive invasion.

The overall score ranges from 2–10, with 2 being the least aggressive and 10 the most aggressive tumour):

Score 2   Atypical adenomatous hyperplasia,

Score 3–4 Low grade, well differentiated,

Score 5–7 Moderately differentiated,

Score 8–10 Poorly differentiated, high grade.

Note: The lowest score that can be attributed on prostatic needle biopsy is 3+3.

Which non-surgical options are available in the management of prostatic cancer?

1. *Active surveillance*: Regular PSA, DRE examinations and repeated prostatic biopsy. This is suitable for men with low-risk prostate cancer whose age and absence of significant co-morbidities would make them eligible for radical treatment if their disease progressed.

2. *Hormone therapy*: Antiandrogen therapy with luteinizing hormone releasing hormone (LHRH) agonists (e.g., Zoladex).

3. Brachytherapy (permanent or temporary implants),

4. External beam radiotherapy.

Which different approaches to radical prostatectomy are utilized?

Open radical prostatectomy –– This may be via a retropubic or perineal approach. In selected cases, where there is a very low risk of seminal vesicle involvement, seminal vesicle sparing may be considered to reduce the risk of cavernous nerve injury. Whilst the retropubic approach is often associated with more significant blood loss, the perineal approach increases the risk of bowel injury and damage to the anal sphincter and does not allow for concomitant removal of the pelvic lymph nodes.

Laparoscopic prostatectomy –– This may be transperitoneal or extraperitoneal. The laparoscopic approach offers improved visualization within the pelvis and reduces overall surgical trauma and blood loss. It has also been reported that improved clearance margins may be attained with laparoscopic and robotic approaches.

Robotic prostatectomy –– The surgeon sits at a remote console performing the procedure via a master–slave robotic system. This technique allows improved mobility of the instruments within the operating space, and offers a benefit by reducing exaggerated instrument motion and hand tremor.

Note: There is currently no robust evidence to say which of these three surgical techniques gives the best outcomes in terms of oncological cure and quality of life.

What are the complications associated with radical prostatectomy?

Immediate –– Bleeding, bowel injury (particularly with perineal approach), ureteral injury.

Early –– Infection, urine leak, urinoma, urinary retention, urinary incontinence, erectile dysfunction.

Late –– Anastomotic stricture, infertility, recurrence.

What are the commonest sites of distant metastasis in prostatic cancer?

Bone (typically sclerotic lesions within the pelvis, femurs or spine), lung, liver.

What is the prevalence of benign prostatic hypertrophy (BPH)?

Reports suggest that symptomatic BPH occurs in up to 8% of men aged 40–49 years and up to 33% at age 60–70 years.

What is the role of transurethral resection of the prostate (TURP)?

This is the most widely used surgical treatment for BPH. In conventional TURP, the resectoscope uses a monopolar electrocautery device with continuous irrigation fluid. Bipolar and laser devices are now available. The resection is usually performed under spinal or general anaesthesia. The patient is placed in the lithotomy position, the resectoscope inserted and an initial cystoscopy performed. The prostatic urethra is then identified and the prostate is resected in a systematic fashion, beginning with the middle lobe, followed by the lateral lobes and finally the apex. Prostatic chippings are sent for histology. Following resection, an irrigating urinary catheter is inserted and continuous irrigation commenced for the first 12–24 hours. The catheter may then be removed once bleeding has sufficiently settled postoperatively.

What are the complications of TURP?

Immediate –– Bleeding, TUR syndrome, clot retention, prostatic capsule perforation.

Early –– Urinary incontinence, failure to improve voiding symptoms.

Late –– Retrograde ejaculation, urethral stenosis, ureteric stenosis (secondary to injury to ureteric orifices), erectile dysfunction, need for repeat TURP.

What is TUR syndrome?

This occurs as a result of absorption of hypotonic irrigation fluid via the prostatic veins and open prostatic sinusoids. The resultant initial rapid intravascular volume expansion may precipitate symptoms of cardiac failure (particularly in patients with impaired left ventricular ejection function). Furthermore, hypotonic fluid absorption leads to systemic hyponatraemia and, if left untreated, may progress to cerebral or pulmonary oedema.

Symptoms and signs include hypertension, confusion, visual disturbances, bradycardia, nausea and vomiting. Where glycine-containing irrigation fluids are used, absorption may also cause glycine intoxication and glycine-induced ammonia intoxication. Clinically, this may manifest as visual disturbances, encephalopathy and seizures.

Testicular torsion and differential diagnoses

At what age does the incidence of testicular torsion peak?

There are two peaks: one in the neonatal period and the second at around age 13–17 years.

What is the aetiology of testicular torsion?

The commonest cause of testicular torsion is secondary to the 'bell clapper' anomaly. This is a congenital anomaly, in which the tunica vaginalis fails to attach to the posterolateral aspect of the testis and instead allows the testicle to move freely within it. 'Intravaginal' torsion of this kind is most commonly seen in adolescence and may occur either spontaneously or secondary to trauma.

'Extravaginal' torsion is usually seen in the neonatal period. The torsion is proximal to the attachment of the tunica vaginalis and occurs in the absence of anatomical abnormality.

What is the classical presentation of testicular torsion?

- Severe, excruciating hemi-scrotal pain (often difficult to examine due to pain),
- Testicular swelling with overlying erythema,
- Nausea or vomiting may be present,
- Absence of urinary symptoms,
- Abnormal 'transverse' lie :the testicle appears to lie higher in the scrotum in the horizontal position,
- Absence of cremasteric reflex on affected side,
- Torsion may be associated with a history of trauma.

What are the differential diagnoses in testicular torsion?

- Epididymitis,
- Orchitis,
- Strangulated inguino-scrotal hernia,
- Torted testicular appendage,
- Acute traumatic injury.

Which imaging modalities may be used to confirm the diagnosis?

It is best practice to proceed immediately (without imaging) to surgical exploration based on clinical findings.

Whilst ultrasound with colour Doppler can be used to demonstrate the absence or reduced blood flow to the affected testicle, it is not usually performed, as it results in delay of definitive treatment (after six hours, irreversible ischaemia begins to occur).

Briefly describe the surgical management of testicular torsion

Where there is a high suspicion of torsion, consent should be obtained and the patient taken to theatre for scrotal exploration as soon as possible. A transverse or median raphe incision (3–5 cm) is made in the scrotum overlying the affected testis. Dissection is made through the dartos and cremasteric layers, to the tunica vaginalis. The testis may then be delivered through the incision. The tunica vaginalis is then incised and any fluid drained. The testis is inspected and manual detorsion is performed. The viability of the affected testis is then assessed once reperfusion has occurred. If the testis appears necrotic or is deemed unviable, orchidectomy is performed. If the testicle appears viable, orchidopexy is performed by three-point fixation, suturing the tunica albuginea to the dartos muscle (non-absorbable suture material may reduce rates of re-torsion although sutures may be felt through the scrotal skin). The contralateral testis is then fixed routinely prior to layered closure of the dartos and the scrotal skin.

Where there is doubt about viability, an incision may be made in the tunica albuginea to confirm lack of arterial flow and ischaemic appearance of the seminiferous tubules. In this case, orchidectomy is required. The testicle is pulled down to expose the distal cord, and the cord structures are identified. Firstly, the vas is clipped and ligated, followed by the testicular vessels. The remainder of the cord is then ligated and transected with careful attention to haemostasis to prevent haematoma formation. The testicle is removed and sent for histology. Finally, the wound may be irrigated prior to closure of the dartos muscle and scrotal skin.

What are the complications associated with emergency scrotal exploration following torsion?

Immediate –– Bleeding and scrotal haematoma, need for orchidectomy.

Early –– Infection, sensation of fixation sutures.

Late –– Reduction in fertility, retorsion.

Testicular malignancies

What are the commonest histological subtypes of testicular tumour?

Germ cell tumours make up 95% of testicular cancers. These are subdivided into:

Seminomatous (~40%)	There is only evidence of seminomatous elements in histological specimen, without elevation of serum α-fetoprotein (as α-FP is secreted by yolk-sac elements of the tumour and therefore by definition this may be non-seminomatous).
Non-seminomatous germ cell tumours (~60%)	Embryonal, teratoma, teratocarcinoma, yolk-sac tumour, choriocarcinoma.

What is the incidence of testicular cancer?

Approximately 6–7 per 100 000 men.

At what age does it commonly occur?

Incidence rates peak at age 25–34 years. There is a second small peak after age 60.

Which aetiological factors have been associated with testicular cancer?

1. Cryptochidism: 2–11× increased risk in men with undescended testes (intra-abdominal > inguinal canal),
2. Genetic: Kleinfelters and Down's syndrome,
3. Family history,
4. *In utero* oestrogen exposure,
5. Infertility.

Which tumour markers are useful in the diagnosis of testicular tumours?

α-Fetoprotein	Raised in approximately 50–70% of non-seminomatous testicular tumours. Produced by yolk-sac cells.
β-Human chorionic gonadotrophin (βHCG)	May be elevated in both seminomatous and non-seminomatous tumours.
Lactate dehydrogenase (LDH)	Can be raised in both seminomatous and non-seminomatous lesions and can be used to monitor disease progression as it provides an indicator of cell turnover and disease burden.

Describe the typical clinical presentation of testicular tumours

The typical finding is of a painless lump felt in the testicle. Rarely, cases may present with an associated hydrocele or testicular pain. Presentation may also be with symptoms of metastatic spread commonly to lungs or retroperitoneum.

What is the staging system?

Staging is based on the TNM system, as proposed by the American Joint Committee against Cancer (AJCC) and the International Union against Cancer (IUC). Primary tumours are assessed as follows:

- **T0** No evidence of primary tumour (Tx means that the tumour cannot be assessed).
- **Tis** Carcinoma *in situ* (intratubular germ cell tumour).
- **T1** The tumour is limited to the epididymis and testis; invasion of the tunica albuginea may be present but there is no invasion into the tunica vaginalis. No evidence of lymphovascular invasion.
- **T2** The tumour is limited to the testis and epididymis and may involve both the tunical albuginea and tunica vaginalis. There is lymphatic or vascular invasion.
- **T3** Spermatic cord invasion is present. There may or may not be lymphovascular invasion.
- **T4** Invasion of the scrotum. There may or may not be lymphovascular invasion.

The TNM staging also includes an 'S', stage which represents the level of the serum tumour markers αFP, LDH and βHCG. These markers are of both prognostic and diagnostic significance.

What are the commonest sites of metastases?

The most common three sites of metastasis are to the lymph nodes, lungs and liver.

What is the prognosis?

The overall cure rate for all stages of seminomatous germ cell tumour is 90%. In stage I disease, the cure rates approach 100%. In non-seminomatous disease, cure rates at stage I are around 95% but drop to around 75% with advanced, stage II–IV disease.

How does orchidectomy for testicular cancer differ from the procedure in acute torsion?

Orchidectomy for malignancy is performed via an inguinal approach with early, high ligation of the spermatic cord at the deep ring. The scrotal approach is contraindicated, as it leaves the inguinal portion of the spermatic cord intact and increases the risk of metastases to scrotal skin and pelvic lymph nodes. Orchidectomy is performed as both a potentially curative and staging procedure without prior needle aspiration or biopsy, due to the risk of seeding of malignant cells.

Circumcision

What are the medical indications for circumcision?

- Phimosis: usually either secondary to congenital adhesions or chronic balanitis),
- Chronic balanitis,
- Recurrent urinary tract infections,
- Irreducible paraphimosis: this is a rare indication when manual reduction is unsuccessful. In this case, a dorsal incision can be made to release the constricting band and a formal circumcision may be performed electively.

Describe the surgical procedure involved in adult circumcision

The procedure is performed under general anaesthesia. After preparing and draping the area, the distal incision is marked at the point of the coronal sulcus. The prepuce is then retracted. After division of any adhesions, the glans is cleaned and the proximal incision marked 5–10 mm from the coronal ridge. The proximal and distal incisions are then made. The foreskin may be resected by either the sleeve or dorsal slit technique. The sleeve technique involves dorsal retraction of the foreskin and dissection of a sleeve of foreskin from Buck's fascia. The dorsal slit technique involves incising the foreskin dorsally between the two incisions. The foreskin is then dissected from the underlying dartos. Haemostasis is achieved and the free edge of skin remaining on the shaft is approximated to the ridge of skin below the corona. Sutures should be interrupted, beginning at the ventral midline approximating both the median raphe and frenulum. The closure is completed with a ring of interrupted absorbable sutures.

What are the complications associated with adult circumcision?

Immediate –– Bleeding, haematoma formation, pain, excision of too much skin.

Early –– Infection, wound dehiscence.

Late –– Stenosis of the urethral meatus, need for repeat circumcision if inadequate excision, altered glans sensitivity and poor cosmetic appearance.

Bibliography

Section 1 Clinical surgery in general

1 Clinical surgery in general

Asbury, S, Mishra, A, and Mokbel, K. M. (2006). *Principles of Operative Surgery: Viva Practice for the MRCS*. Radcliffe Publishing.

Ethicon, Inc. (2011). www.ethicon360.com.

Neudecker, J., Sauerland, S., Neugebauer, E. *et al.* (2002). The European Association for Endoscopic Surgery: clinical practice guideline on the pneumoperitoneum for laparoscopic surgery. *Surg. Endosc.*, **16**, 1121–43.

Whelan, R. L., Fleshman, J. and Fowler, D. L. (2005). *The SAGES Manual of Perioperative Care in Minimally Invasive Surgery*. Springer.

Section 2 Thorax

2 Applied surgical anatomy

Cohn, L. H. (2008). *Cardiac Surgery in the Adult*. McGraw-Hill Medical.

Ellis, H. (2006). *Clinical Anatomy: Applied Anatomy for Students and Junior Doctors*. Blackwell Science.

Sinnatamby, C. S. and Last, R. J. (2006). *Last's Anatomy: Regional and Applied*. Churchill Livingstone.

3 Applied surgical physiology: cardiovascular

Kanani, M. and Elliott, M. (2004). *Applied Surgical Physiology Vivas*. Cambridge University Press.

Nichols, W. W. (2005). Clinical measurement of arterial stiffness obtained from noninvasive pressure waveforms. *Am. J. Hypertens.*, **18**(1 Pt 2), 3S–10S.

Silbernagl, S. and Despopoulos, A. (2009). *Color Atlas of Physiology*. Thieme.

4 Surgical approaches to the chest

Dürrleman, N. and Massard G. (2006). Elective anterior and posterior thoracotomies. *MMCTS*, **2006**(0810), 1446.

Dürrleman, N. and Massard, G. (2006). Antero-lateral thoracotomy. *MMCTS*, **2006**(0810), 1859.

Dürrleman, N. and Massard, G. (2006). Clamshell and hemiclamshell incisions. *MMCTS*, **2006**(0810), 1867.

Kanani, M. (2002). *Surgical Critical Care Vivas*. Cambridge University Press.

Sundaresan, S. (2003) Left thoracoabdominal incision. *Oper. Techn. Thorac. Cardiovasc. Surg.*, **8**(2), 71–85.

5 The mediastinum and diaphragm

Knipp, B. S., Deeb, G. M., Prager, R. L. *et al.* (2007). A contemporary analysis of outcomes for operative repair of type A aortic dissection in the United States. *Surgery*, **142**(4), 524–8.

Trimarchi, S., Nienaber, C. A., Rampoldi, V. *et al.* (2005). Contemporary results of surgery in acute type A aortic dissection: the International Registry of Acute Aortic Dissection experience. *J. Thorac. Cardiovasc. Surg.*, **129**(1), 112–22.

6 The breast: benign and malignant disease

Burstein, H. J. and Winer, E. P. (2000). Primary care for survivors of breast cancer. *New Engl. J. Med.*, **343**(15), 1086–94.

Hartmann, L. C., Sellers, T. A., Frost, M. H. *et al.* (2005). Benign breast disease and the risk of breast cancer. *New Engl. J. Med.*, **353**(3), 229–37.

Hussain, M. and Cunnick, G. H. (2011). Management of lobular carcinoma *in-situ* and atypical lobular hyperplasia of the breast – a review. *Eur. J. Surg. Oncol.*, **37**(4), 279–89.

National Institute for Health and Clinical Excellence (2009). *Early and Locally Advanced Breast Cancer: Full Guidelines [CG80]*. National Institute for Health and Clinical Excellence.

Serletti, J. M. (2006). Breast reconstruction with the TRAM flap: pedicled and free. *J. Surg. Oncol.*, **94**(6), 532–7.

Section 3 Trunk

7 Applied surgical anatomy

Ellis, H. (2006). *Clinical Anatomy: Applied Anatomy for Students and Junior Doctors*. Blackwell Science.

Sinnatamby, C. S. and Last, R. J. (2006). *Last's Anatomy: Regional and Applied*. Churchill Livingstone.

8 Applied surgical physiology

Kanani, M. and Elliott, M. (2004). *Applied Surgical Physiology Vivas*. Cambridge University Press.

Silbernagl, S. and Despopoulos, A. (2009). *Color Atlas of Physiology*. Thieme.

9 The abdominal wall

Sakorafas, G. H., *et al.* (2001). Open tension free repair of inguinal hernias; the Lichtenstein technique. *BMC Surg.*, **1**, 3.

10 The abdominal aorta and abdominal aortic aneurysms

Ailawadi, G., Knipp, B. S., Lu, G. *et al.* (2003). A nonintrinsic regional basis for increased infrarenal aortic MMP-9 expression and activity. *J. Vas. Surg.* **37**(5), 1059–66.

Alexander, D. J., James, P. J., Vowden, P., Abbott, C. R., Doig, R. L. (1992). Syphilitic aortitis with rupture of the infrarenal aorta; seen and not forgotten. *Eur. J. Vasc. Surg.*, **6**(1), 98–100.

Beard, J. D. and Gaines, P. A. (2009). *Vascular and Endovascular Surgery: A Companion to Specialist*

Surgical Practice. Elsevier Health Sciences.

Cronenwett, J. L., Johnston, W. and Rutherford, R. B. (2010). *Rutherford's Vascular Surgery.* Saunders.

United Kingdom EVAR Trial Investigators (2005). Endovascular aneurysm repair versus open repair in patients with abdominal aortic aneurysm (EVAR trial 1): randomised controlled trial. *Lancet,* **365**(9478), 2179–86.

United Kingdom EVAR Trial Investigators (2005). Endovascular aneurysm repair and outcome in patients unfit for open repair of abdominal aortic aneurysm (EVAR trial 2): randomised controlled trial. *Lancet,* **365**(9478), 2187–92.

Zarins, C. K., Gewertz, B. L., Kraus Biomédical and Hirsh, K. (2007). *Atlas de chirurgie vasculaire.* Elsevier Masson.

11 The oesophagus, stomach and small bowel

Fuccio, L., Minardi, M. E., Zagari, R. M. *et al.* (2007). Meta-analysis: duration of first-line proton-pump inhibitor based triple therapy for *Helicobacter pylori* eradication. *Ann. Intern. Med.,* **147**(8), 553–62.

Malfertheiner, P., Chan, F. K. and McColl, K. E. (2009). Peptic ulcer disease. *Lancet,* **374**(9699), 1449–61.

Rockall, T. A., Logan, R. F., Devlin, H. B. and Northfield, T. C. (1996). Risk assessment after acute upper gastrointestinal haemorrhage. *Gut,* **38**(3), 316–21.

12 The liver, biliary tree and pancreas

Bahra, M. and Neuhaus, P. (2010). Pancreas: is there still a role for total pancreatectomy? *Nat. Rev. Gastroenterol. Hepatol.* **7**(2), 72–4.

Bollen, T. L, van Santvoort, H. C., Besselink, M. G, *et al.* (2008). The Atlanta classification of acute pancreatitis revisited. *Br. J. Surg,* **95**(1), 6–21.

Burton, F., Alkaade, S. Collins, D. *et al.* (2011). Use and perceived effectiveness of non-analgesic medical therapies for chronic pancreatitis in the United States. *Aliment. Pharm. Therap.,* **33**(1), 149–59.

Chen, W. X., Zhang, W.-F., Li, B., et al. (2006). Clinical manifestations of patients with chronic pancreatitis. *Hepatobiliary Pancreat. Dis. Int.,* **5**(1), 133–7.

Frossard, J-L, Steer, M. L. and Pastor, C. M. (2008). Acute pancreatitis. *Lancet,* **371**(9607), 143–52.

Gourgiotis, S. Kocher, H. M., Solaini, L. *et al.* (2008). Gallbladder cancer. *Am. J. Surg.,* **196**(2), 252–64.

Loos, M, Kleeff, J., Friess, H. and Büchler, M. W. (2008). Surgical treatment of pancreatic cancer. *Ann. NY Acad. Sci.,* **1138**, 169–80.

Reddy, S. K., Tyler, D. S., Pappas, T. N. and Clary, B. M. (2007). Extended resection for pancreatic adenocarcinoma. *Oncologist.* **12**(6), 654–63.

Shaffer, E. A. (2006). Epidemiology of gallbladder stone disease. *Best Pract. Res. Cl. Ga.,* **20**(6), 981–96.

UK Working Party on Acute Pancreatitis (2005). UK guidelines for the management of acute pancreatitis. *Gut*, **54**(Suppl. 3), 1–9.

13 The spleen: splenic trauma and splenectomy

Forsythe, R. M., Harbrecht, B. G. and Peitzman, A. B. (2006). Blunt splenic trauma. *Scand. J. Surg.*, **95**(3), 146–51.

Franklin, G. A. and Casos, S. R. (2006). Current advances in the surgical approach to abdominal trauma. *Injury*, **37**(12), 1143–56.

Harbrecht, B. G. (2005). Is anything new in adult blunt splenic trauma? *Am. J. Surg.*, **190**(2), 273–8.

Holden A. (2008). Abdomen – interventions for solid organ injury. *Injury*, **39**(11), 1275–89.

Lucas, C. E. (1991). Splenic trauma. Choice of management. *Ann. Surg.*, **213**(2), 98–112.

Renzulli, P., Hostettler, A., Schoepfer, A. M., Gloor, B. and Candinas, D. (2009). Systematic review of atraumatic splenic rupture. *Br. J. Surg.*, **96**(10), 1114–21.

14 The large bowel

Audisio, R. A., Geraghty, J. G. and Longo, W. E. (2001). *Modern Management of Cancer of the Rectum*. Springer.

Canon, C. L. (2008). Is there still a role for double-contrast barium enema examination? *Clin. Gastroenterol. Hepatol.*, **6**(4), 389–92.

Chowdhury, F. U., Shah, N., Scarsbrook, A. F. and Bradley, K. M. (2010). [^{18}F]FDG PET/CT imaging of colorectal cancer: a pictorial review. *Postgrad. Med. J.*, **86**(1013), 174–82.

Duffy, M. J., van Dalen, A., Haglund, C. *et al.* (2007). Tumour markers in colorectal cancer: European Group on Tumour Markers (EGTM) guidelines for clinical use. *Eur. J. Cancer*, **43**(9), 1348–60.

Eng, C. (2010). The evolving role of monoclonal antibodies in colorectal cancer: early presumptions and impact on clinical trial development. *Oncologist*, **15**(1), 73–84.

Half, E., Bercovich, D. and Rozen, P. (2009). Familial adenomatous polyposis. *Orphanet. J. Rare Dis.*, **4**, 22.

Hwang, J. M. and Varma, M. G. (2008). Surgery for inflammatory bowel disease. *World J. Gastroenterol.*, **14**(17), 2678–90.

Leslie, A., Carey, F. A., Pratt, N. R. and Steele, R. J. (2002). The colorectal adenoma-carcinoma sequence. *Br. J. Surg.*, **89**(7), 845–60.

Lombardi, L., Morelli, F., Cinieri, S. *et al.* (2010). Adjuvant colon cancer chemotherapy: where we are and where we'll go. *Cancer Treat. Rev.*, **36**(Supplement 3), S34–S41.

National Cancer Intelligence Network. (1996–2002). Survival from Colorectal Cancer by Stage. www.ncin.org.uk.

Ng, S. C. and Kamm, M. A. (2009). Therapeutic strategies for the management of ulcerative colitis. *Inflamm. Bowel Dis.*, **15**(6), 935–50.

NHS (2011). *Bowel Cancer Screening: The Facts*. www.cancerscreening.nhs.uk/bowel/index.html.

Skandalakis, L. J., Skandalakis, J. E. and Skandalakis, P. N. (2009). *Surgical Anatomy and Technique: a Pocket Manual*. Springer.

Vasen, H. F. (2005). Clinical description of the Lynch syndrome [hereditary nonpolyposis colorectal cancer (HNPCC)]. *Fam. Cancer*, **4**(3), 219–25.

15 The rectum and anus

Acheson, A. G. and Scholefield, J. H. (2008). Management of haemorrhoids. *BMJ*, **336**(7640), 380–3.

Chintapatla, S., Safarani, N., Kumar, S. and Haboubi, N. (2003). Sacrococcygeal pilonidal sinus: historical review, pathological insight and surgical options. *Tech. Coloproctol.*, **7**(1), 3–8.

Collins, E. E. and Lund, J. N. (2007). A review of chronic anal fissure management. *Tech. Coloproctol.*, **11**(3), 209–23.

Deeba, S., Aziz, O., Sains, P. S. and Darzi, A. (2008). Fistula-in-ano: advances in treatment. *Am. J. Surg.*, **196**(1), 95–9.

Giordano, P., Overton, J., Madeddu, F., Zaman, S. and Gravante, G. (2009). Transanal hemorrhoidal dearterialization: a systematic review. *Dis. Colon. Rectum*, **52**(9), 1665–71.

Hardy, A., Chan, C. L. and Cohen, C. R. (2005). The surgical management of haemorrhoids: a review. *Dig. Surg.*, **22**(1–2), 26–33.

NICE (2007). *Closure of Anorectal Fistula Using a Suturable Bioprosthetic Plug (Interventional Procedures Overview)*. National Institute for Health and Clinical Excellence.

Ratto, C., Donisi, L., Parello, A., Litta, F. and Doglietto, G. B. (2010). Evaluation of transanal hemorrhoidal dearterialization as a minimally invasive therapeutic approach to hemorrhoids. *Dis. Colon Rectum*, **53**(5), 803–11.

Shabbir, J., Chaudhary, B. N. and Britton, D. C. (2011). Management of sacrococcygeal pilonidal sinus disease: a snapshot of current practice. *Int. J. Colorectal Dis.* (14 March 2011), 1–2.

Uronis, H. E. and Bendell, J. C. (2007). Anal cancer: an overview. *Oncologist*, **12**(5), 524–34.

16 The kidneys and genitourinary system

Andriole, G. L. (2009). Prostate cancer risk: overview of the disease, predictive factors, and potential targets for risk reduction. Introduction. *Urology*. **73**(5 Suppl), S1–3.

Baazeem, A. and Elhilali, M. M. (2008). Surgical management of benign prostatic hyperplasia: current evidence. *Nat. Clin. Pract. Urol.*, **5**(10), 540–9.

Billingham, R. P., Kobashi, K. C. and Peters, W. A. (2009). *Reoperative Pelvic Surgery*. Springer.

Bjartell, A. (2006). Words of wisdom. The 2005 International Society of Urological Pathology (ISUP) consensus conference on Gleason grading of prostatic carcinoma. *Eur. Urol.*, **49**(4), 758–9.

Carver, B. and Sheinfeld, J. (2005). Germ cell tumors of the testis. *Ann. Surg. Oncol.*, **12**(11), 871–80.

Dickinson, S. I. (2010) Premalignant and malignant prostate lesions: pathologic review. *Cancer Control.* **17**(4), 214–22.

Epstein, J. I., Allsbrook, W. C., Jr., Amin, M. B. and Egevad, L. L. (2005). The 2005 International Society of Urological Pathology (ISUP) consensus conference on Gleason grading of prostatic carcinoma. *Am. J. Surg. Pathol.*, **29**(9), 1228–42.

Gjertson, C. K. and Albertsen, P. C. (2011). Use and Assessment of PSA in prostate cancer. *Med. Clin. N. Am.*, **95**(1), 191–200.

Gori, S., Porrozzi, S., Roila, F. *et al.* (2005). Germ cell tumours of the testis. *Crit. Rev. Oncol. Hemat.*, **53**(2), 141–64.

Hashim, H., Abrams, P., Dmochowski, R. and Dmochowski, R. R. (2008). *Handbook of Office Urological Procedures*. Springer.

Helpap, B. and Egevad, L. (2009). Modified Gleason grading. An updated review. *Histol. Histopathol.*, **24**(5), 661–6.

Kapoor, S. (2008). Testicular torsion: a race against time. *Int. J. Clin. Pract.*, **62**(5), 821–7.

Meraney, A. M., Haese, A., Palisaar, J. *et al.* (2005). Surgical management of prostate cancer: Advances based on a rational approach to the data. *Eur. J. Cancer*, **41**(6), 888–907.

Preminger, G. M., Tiselius, H.-G., Assimos, D. G. *et al.* (2007). 2007 guideline for the management of ureteral calculi. *J. Urol.*, **178**(6), 2418–34.

Sexton, W. J., Wiegand, L. R., Correa, J. J. *et al.* (2010). Bladder cancer: a review of non-muscle invasive disease. *Cancer Control*, **17**(4), 256–68.

Stenzl, A., Cowan, N. C., De Santis, M. *et al.* (2011). Treatment of muscle-invasive and metastatic bladder cancer: update of the EAU guidelines. *Eur. Urol.*, **59**(6), 1009–18.

Worcester, E. M. and Coe, F. L. (2010). Clinical practice. Calcium kidney stones. *N. Engl. J. Med.*, **363**(10), 954–63.

Index

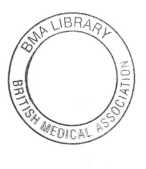